Tea for Menopause.

A little cup goes a long way.

Anita Williams

Qualified Naturopath, Nutritionist,

Mother, Grandmother

&

Herbal Tea Lover.

Tea for Menopause

Disclaimer

This book is not to be used as a substitute for professional medical care and treatment. The ultimate decision concerning care should be between you and your health care professional. The information in this book is given with no guarantees on the part of the author or publisher. Every care has been taken to ensure the accuracy of information in this book. However, if there are any errors or omissions, if informed, corrections will be made in any future editions.

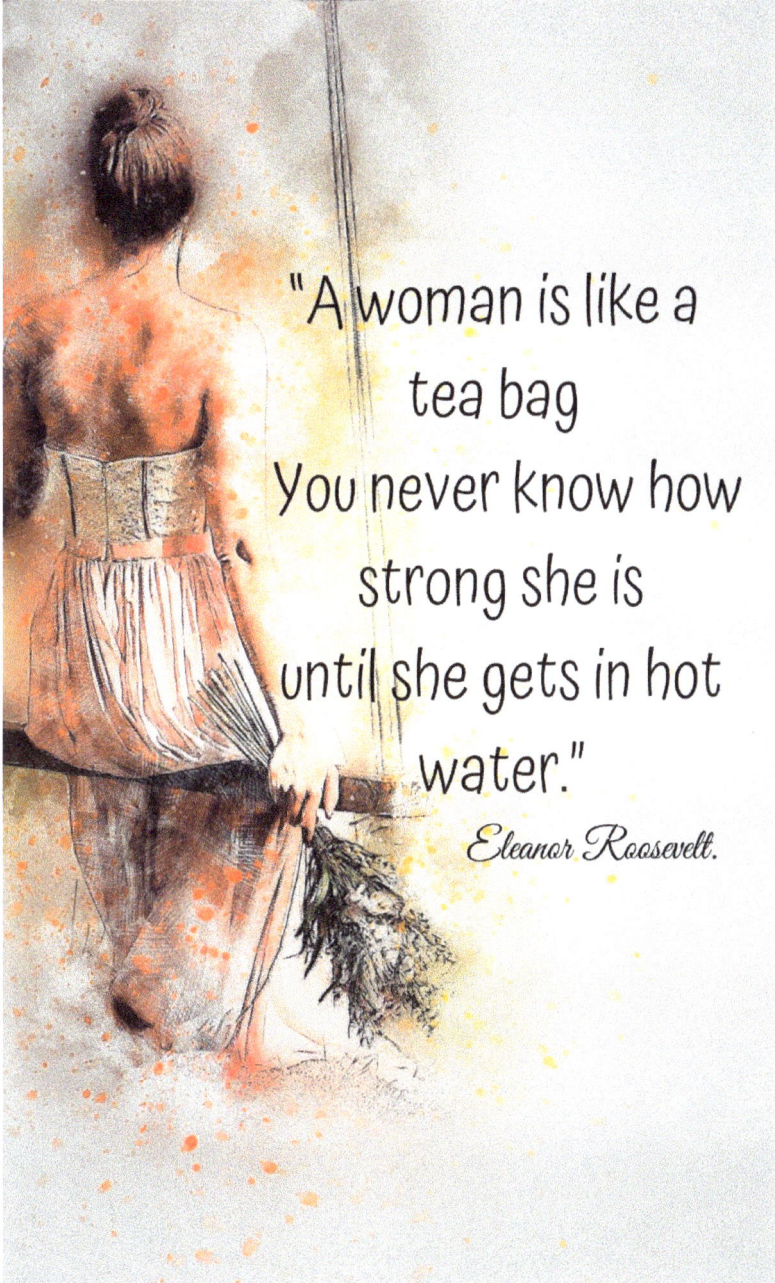

"A woman is like a
tea bag
You never know how
strong she is
until she gets in hot
water."
Eleanor Roosevelt.

Message from the author

If God brings you to it, he will help you walk through it. It is a blessing to reach the age of wisdom and for many women the reaching of menopause marks the reaching of wisdom. It certainly has for me.

Have you ever noticed how some people try to make life more complicated than it needs to be? It seems to me that we are here on earth for such a short time and that we should live life to its fullest. To gain the best experience here, we need our bodies to be functioning optimally and the desire to see women enjoy their experience here on earth is what inspired me to write this book.

This book is designed to be a tool to help women transition through menopause. I hope it is a book that will be passed down from mothers to daughters, through generations, with each adding their personal notations. For as no two women experience the same menstrual cycle or birth story, no two women will experience the same transition through perimenopause into menopause and beyond.

Reaching menopause is a milestone to be celebrated. Mindset is important when dealing with change and menopause is a time of change. Use this time of transition to assess and celebrate what you have done. You are fabulous and plan for the years ahead.

I have investigated over one hundred different teas, which may be combined to enhance outcomes, that have been used traditionally and some which have scientific evidence to assist women transition through menopause and live rich full lives.

Understanding which teas have the potential to assist you transition through menopause is what this book is about. Keep notes in the back of the book so the women of tomorrow may see how women of today used teas to assist with menopause. Pass this knowledge on to the women of tomorrow.

May each woman who reads this book be blessed with the joy and fulfilment that comes from knowing who you are and where you belong!

May God bless you with good health in abundance!

Acknowledgements

As this is the first book I have ever attempted, I naively thought it would be a quick process. This was far from the truth and along the way I have been blessed to have the support and assistance of some wonderful people who I would like to thank.

Much love to my family for their support and assistance through the process of writing and publishing this book.

Heartfelt thanks to;

Mary-Leigh Scheerhoorn for all her assistance with the photo shoot.

Megan Cartwright for her assistance with the editing, photo shoot and loving support throughout the production of this book.

Nathaniel Deering for technical support and production of book covers.

Rose Flannery for her assistance with editing and participation in photo shoot.

Kyra Howearth for her assistance in providing me with the herbal photos.

To my friend Mel Combe for always being willing to listen and support.

Tammy Guest, my mentor, for providing guidance and continuous positive encouragement.

Cover photo by Mary-Leigh Scheerhoorn.

Tea for Menopause.

A little cup goes a long way.

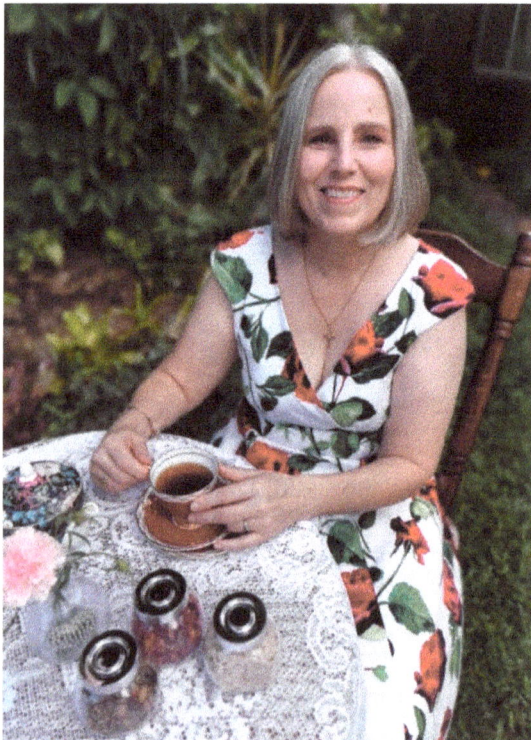

Contents

Section 1

What is menopause?

How do tea and menopause come together?

What is tea?

Properties of tea.

Buying the right tea.

How to store your tea.

Water temperature.

Section 2

Tea Index

Section 3

Tea blends

Tea for Menopause

Section 1

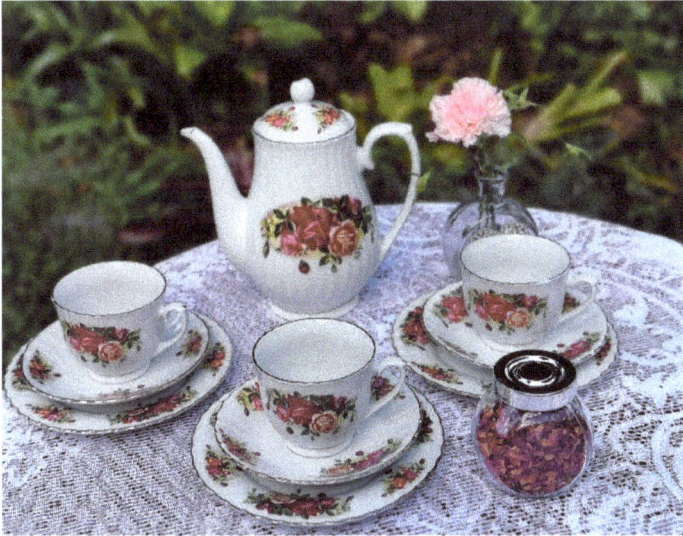

What is Menopause?

Menopause is only one day in your life. It is the day one year after your last menstrual cycle. However, when most people and articles talk about menopause, they are usually including perimenopause and sometimes post menopause, the years after the one day of menopause. For some women the symptoms of menopause have been known to last for as long as ten years.

Perimenopause the pre-runner to menopause is the time when women often experience what is referred to as menopausal symptoms.

Depending on the source the number of symptoms for menopause may slightly differ but in this book 47 symptoms are investigated to determine which teas may be of benefit to you as you go through the menopausal transition.

Menopausal transition occurs because you have come to the end of your reproductive years. Once you have reached menopause you have no eggs left inside your ovaries. During the perimenopausal period (the average length of perimenopause is four years) hormones levels fluctuate and symptoms may be experienced.

15-20% of women go through menopausal transition without any symptoms. 15-20% of women have horrendous symptoms that are debilitating and impacts their life terribly. For the other 60-70% the symptoms and duration vary. It is for this group that tea is a great option. Not to say that for those with severe symptoms tea won't assist, it just may not be enough on its own. It is important to know the symptoms of menopause, know your treatment options, both natural and allopathic (medical intervention to treat a condition via the use of medication or surgery) and gather all the information you can to make the best decision for your health.

How do tea and menopause come together?

Historically women worldwide have used tea to address the symptoms of menopause. Tea is relatively cheap; it can be made from plants in your own garden or sourced from nature. This process is called wild crafting. Today tea can be purchased from shops both physical and online.

The beauty of living in the 21ST century is that the world of plants is open to us. The internet allows us to access may different varieties of plants and teas. The trick is to know which tea is best for you and to ensure the quality of the tea is of a high standard.

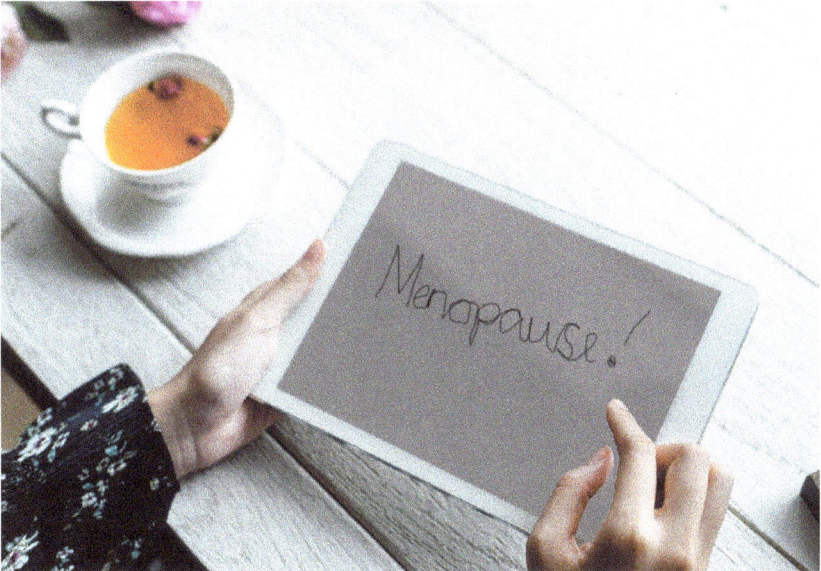

What is tea?

Definition

Defining tea isn't quite as simple as one first thinks. The first thing that comes to mind is a steaming hot cup of tea which was made from tea leaves, which was grown on a tea bush which may or may not have had additional flavours added to it.

A cup of tea is usually made from tea leaves, but can also be made from the fruit, bark, stem, flower or root of a plants.

The Tea plant Camellia sinensis gives us the major types of tea;

- Green tea - unfermented
- Yellow tea - lightly fermented
- Oolong - semi fermented
- Black tea - fully fermented
- White tea may be simply dried or lightly fermented.

Herbal tea comes from a variety of plants and trees which are used worldwide to assist women with their menopausal transition. Some tea blends combine tea from the *camellia sinensis* plant with other herbs and flavouring agents. It is important that you read the labels when buying tea to be sure you are getting real ingredients not artificial flavourings and sweeteners which may be made in a laboratory and have no additional benefit.

Properties of tea

Polyphenols are compounds which contains more than one phenolic hydroxyl group in their chemical makeup. They are accredited with providing antioxidant, antiviral and anti-inflammatory actions. There are more than 500 different polyphenols and collectively they are referred to as phytochemicals. Polyphenols include catechins, which are the most studied of the constituents in tea. Tea also contains the polyphenol theaflavins. Theaflavins occur in tea due to enzymatic oxidation. Laboratory studies and animal testing of theaflavin have identified it as being one of the constituents in tea responsible for providing antiviral and anti-cancer properties, as well as making it a potent antioxidant.

Flavonoids are a group of phytonutrients; chemicals found in most fruit and vegetables and are some of the world's healthiest foods. Flavonoids are the pigments in plants that give them their vibrant colours. There are over 6000 flavonoids. They are accredited as being great antioxidants. Flavonoids in some cases have been found to be anti-cancer, anti-diabetic and may assist with muscle pain and improve wellbeing. Flavonoids are water soluble which means you can get the benefit from having them as tea.

As you will have gathered the science of tea is expansive. This book is about helping you chose the right tea for you not explaining the science. However, there are a few things that you should be aware of;

1. Tannins are another water-soluble polyphenol found in tea and some herbal teas. They have a bitter taster and have the capacity to bind to protein. This ability is useful in cases of diarrhoea where the high tannins content of black tea binds with the protein in the gut creating a barrier reducing water loss. Tannins also inhibit the absorption of iron. Women who are taking iron supplements or who must increase iron levels should consider drinking teas high in tannins one to two hours either side of taking supplements or eating your iron rich foods.

2. Aroma of tea is due to aromatic volatiles. In tea from the *camellia sinensis* plant more than 600 volatiles are identified as influencing the aroma and flavour of tea. In herbal tea each herb has its own aromatic volatiles that influence the aroma and flavour. Many of these herbs are

used to make essential oils and you may be tempted to use an essential oil to flavour your tea. Do not do this. Essential oils are extremely concentrated and if ingested could cause harm or be fatal. For example, it takes approximately 242,000 rose petals to make 5ml of rose oil. You would never put that number of rose petals in your tea.

3. Caffeine

Some teas may contain caffeine. Caffeine is a stimulant. It works by stimulating the central nervous system. For some people caffeine may impact negatively on their menopausal transition. Caffeine may interfere with some people's ability to sleep, increase anxiety symptoms and some women find it triggers migraines.

Oxidation

Oxidation is the loss of an electron during a reaction by an atom, molecule or ion. When plants are picked, crushed or damaged oxidation takes place. When tea is oxidized, polyphenols reactions start this is carried out by enzymes within the leaf reacting to oxygen. This converts catechins into other constituents such as thearubigins and theaflavins which each potentiate certain health benefits. It also activates the breakdown of fats, proteins and plant pigments which results in different flavours and aromas of the tea.

Oxidation process of Camellia sinensis to produce different teas:

- Green tea - unoxidized
- White tea - wilted and unoxidized
- Yellow tea - unwilted and unoxidized but allowed to yellow.
- Oolong - 10-85% oxidized
- Black tea - fully oxidized

Herbal teas are usually produced by collecting the herbs, stem, flower, fruit or bark and drying. They do not normally go through an oxidation process in manufacturing.

Why people drink tea

People drink tea for many reasons. It may be part of a cultural ceremony, a festival or religious celebration. People use tea to treat a variety of different ailments. Others drink tea to warm or cool the body and to enjoy the flavours.

It is generally recommended that you drink no more than 3-4 cups of tea a day to gain optimal health benefits. This may differ depending on the type of tea you are drinking and your current state of health. If you wish to consume large amounts of any tea or if you have a health condition, please consult with a health care professional before consuming large volumes of tea.

Which tea to buy?

Getting the name right

It is important to get the name right when buying tea and herbs to use in teas. As some plants are similarly named or have a common name but have not been shown to have any benefit when treating symptoms associated with menopause.

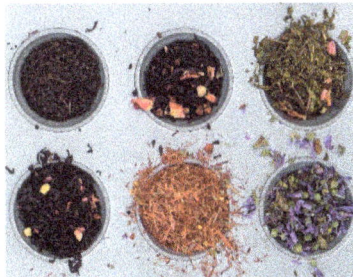

Organic

Is it worth spending the extra money to purchase organic tea? Put simply the answer is yes. While many teas have been identified as having anti-carcinogenic properties many of the pesticides used to produce these teas have been proven to be possible carcinogens.

There are more than 300 different pesticides used on tea crops, and they are not the only way that tea may be contaminated. Contamination can come from the soil; for example, too much arsenic in the soil may result in the plant having high arsenic levels which would then be passed on to consumers. Air pollution and sprays from neighbouring fields may also impact on the quality of tea.

Organic teas have come to the forefront of tea consumption in the last decade. Organic tea is produced without the use of chemical fertilizers, herbicides or pesticides. Instead natural organic matter is added to nourish the soil.

There are many bodies that certify tea as organic. Some require 100% organic ingredients; others go down as low as 70% organic ingredients. Product labels will advise of organic content. Remember 70% organic is more advantageous than 0% organic.

If you are about to make your own herbal teas from your garden or a friend's garden, you will have greater knowledge of growing processes and environmental impact on your tea. You also have the benefit of fresh produce.

After reading this book you may decide to plant a few herbs to assist you with your menopausal tea journey.

Storage

What to avoid when storing tea. You want to avoid getting your tea wet or moist, so an airtight container is recommended. Tea is better stored in large amounts as this allows for reduced exposure of the leaves to the air.

Store your tea away from heat. A cool dark pantry is ideal. Herbal teas are the same, store them in airtight containers. Ceramics or tins are ideal for long term storage keeping then safe from moisture, light and strong odours.

Tea may also be kept in the freezer, but once thawed it is best to use and not refrozen. Refreezing may result in the structure and flavour being compromised that thus you end up with a lower quality tea.

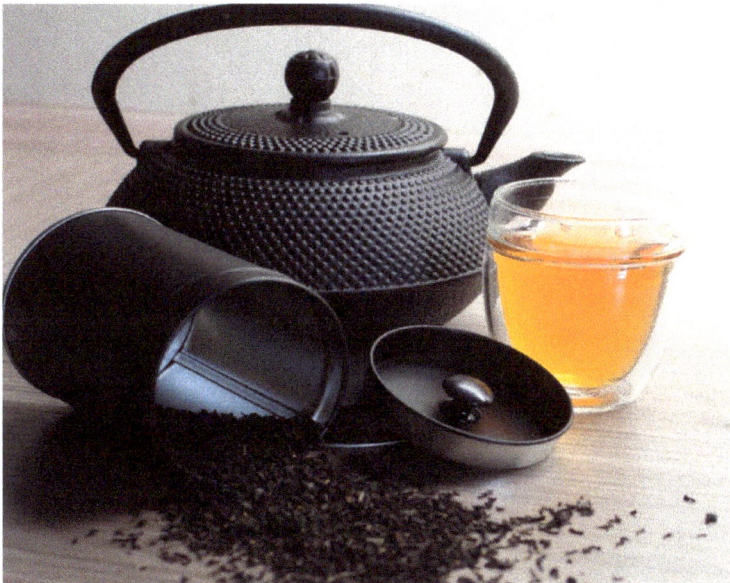

How to make tea

Water temperature

A "Tea Sommelier" is someone who has studied and is trained in all things tea and they would be the perfect person to contact if you are greatly interested in the finer points of tea making. For this book we are looking at the basics of making tea with the aim to assist women transitioning through menopause.

That being said I still will touch on some of the important points of tea making. One of those is water temperature.

The number one rule is never boil the water. Now most people aren't going to stand there and watch the water to ensure it doesn't boil, but true tea lovers may. Today we have the luxury of being able to purchase kettles that bring the water to the right temperature for the tea you are making.

In this book you will see the term off the boil, this is just before the water boils, where bubbles are coming up but not yet boiling, if you don't want the hassle of watching your water, you can boil the water and let it cool for a couple of minutes. To a tea sommelier this would not be an acceptable practice as the water may be altered, but for the general person this would be okay. For the menopausal woman experiencing symptoms the boiling of water may not be a high priority, so just get that tea made and start drinking ladies. The basic fact is that each tea has an ideal temperature to produce the best flavour and ensure the constituents are in peak condition for our bodies to use. If the water is too hot it can burn the leaves, this is more prominent in the unfermented unoxidized teas such as white, yellow and green. You may wish to pour the water into the cup before adding the leaves or pour the water down the insides of the tea pot rather than over the leaves, just allowing it to cool slightly before touching the leaves. If the water is to hot the flavour of the tea may become more bitter, astringent and unbalanced. If the water is too cold the flavours and constituents may not be released fully and you may not get the maximum benefit.

Different tea companies suggest slightly different temperatures for making tea but here is a general guide:

- White tea 70-80 degrees Celsius
- Yellow tea 79 degrees Celsius
- Green tea 70-80 degrees Celsius
- Oolong tea 80-90 degrees Celsius
- Black tea 95 degrees Celsius
- Herbal tea 90-95 degrees Celsius.

Different sources will provide you with slightly different ranges, but they all suggest you keep it below boiling. So, when you read the How to brew where it says boiling water, remember you want your water just below boiling. For optimum tea use fresh water for every pot you make.

Infusions

How to make an Herbal Infusion

An infusion is a drink that is made by steeping. Steeping is when you soak your tea in water to extract flavour, colour or soften. To gain therapeutic benefits and to extract flavour tea leaves and herbs are most commonly soaked in hot water. There are a few options for making an infusion of tea and herbal teas.

Option 1. Tea pot.

First, start by warming your tea pot with some boiled water. Swirl it around and tip the water out. Place tea into the pot. A tea infuser may be included, if not you may wish to strain your tea as you pour it.

Option 2. Single cup infusion.

If a tea pot seems wasteful for single use, a tea bag or a tea ball can be used. Simply place your tea in the tea ball or bag, pop it in you cup with hot water and steep.

You can keep your infusion to drink later as iced tea or choose to make it into a jelly.

Option 3. Cold Infusion.

 This tea is made by using water at room temperature. It is often used with mucilaginous herbs as water can extract the polysaccharides from the herbs. To make a cold infusion you use a jar or container with a sealed lid. Place the required amount of herb in the jar, this will vary depending on the herb being used. Fill jar with water and let steep, this may range from a few hours to a day depending on herb being used.

Making tea into jelly is achieved by adding gelatine or Agar Agar and placing in the refrigerator to set.

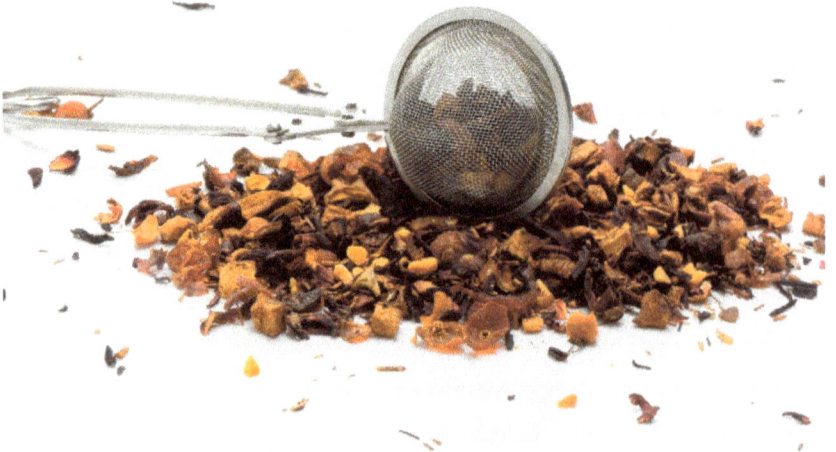

Decoctions

Basics

How to make an Herbal Decoction

Use one to four teaspoon of each herb per cup of cold water. This will vary from herb to herb. You will find these amounts in the how to brew section of each ingredient.

Place cold water and herb/s in a saucepan.

Place saucepan on heat and bring to a gentle boil.

Place a lid on the saucepan and gently simmer for 10-20 minutes. Times can vary depending on herbs being used.

For herbal teas with volatile oil components steep with the lid on to retain optimum benefits.

Remove from heat and allow to cool to drinking temperature.

Store in sealed container, preferably glass for up to 48 hrs in the refrigerator.

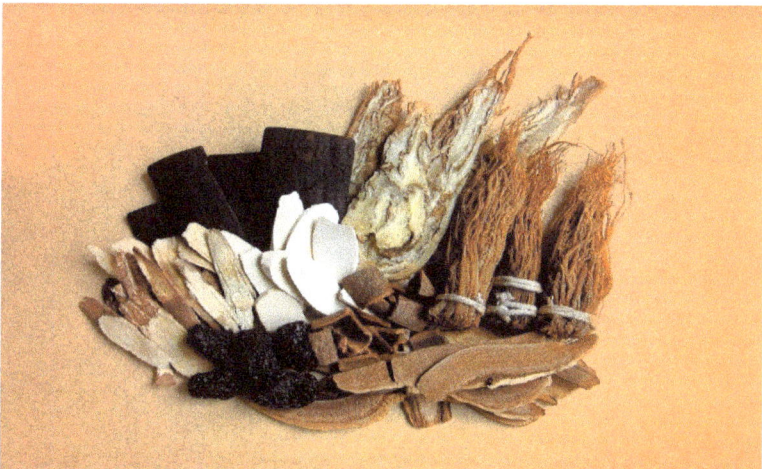

Additives

Throughout history people have added things to alter the tastes of tea. The inclusion of different herbs and spices change the flavour. I would suggest you use other flavourings, herbs and spices that also address menopausal symptoms. There are many options covered later in this book. Ginger and citrus are my personal favourites.

Generally herbal teas are consumed without milk. Some people prefer their tea sweetened. I would advise to try them unsweetened for optimum health. Consult with your natural health care provider about the use of sweeteners.

The bitter flavour of many herbs is salutary and by adding sweeteners you may neutralize these benefits.

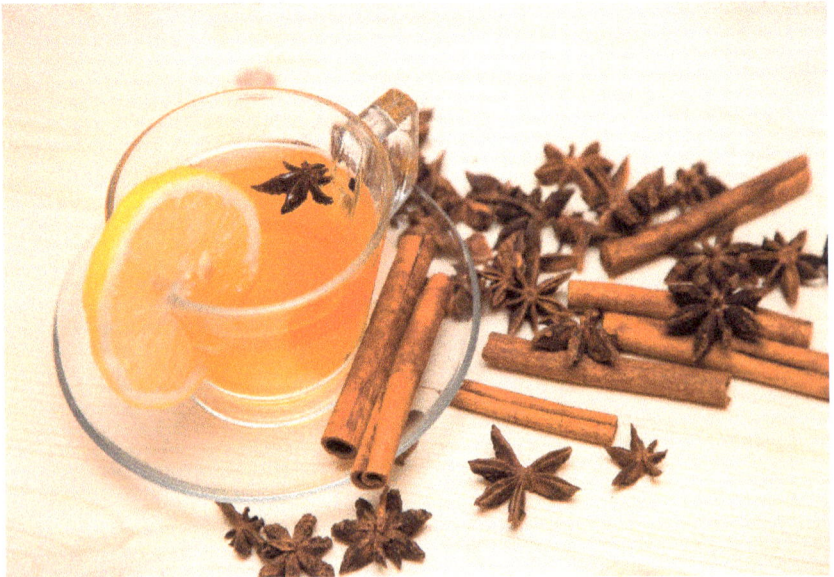

Cold teas

Cold teas may be prepared using any method. They are of great assistance to menopausal women who are feeling hot and bothered. They are fantastic for those living in hot climates.

To make cold tea simply make your hot tea and refrigerate. You may also wish to freeze some of your tea to add as ice cubes. There is no hard or fast rule to how to make cold tea and there are many different options. General pointers would be keeping your tea covered and refrigerated, you don't want it to take on flavours of other foods in your fridge. If you aren't going to consume your tea in 48 hrs turn it into ice cubes.

Try not to add to much if any sweetener. Some recipes call for a lot of sugar, try to avoid these as you may lose the benefit of your tea. Instead use rose petals, violets, mint and lemon balm which have a naturally sweet taste. You can even add these to your ice cubes for a great effect in your tea when serving.

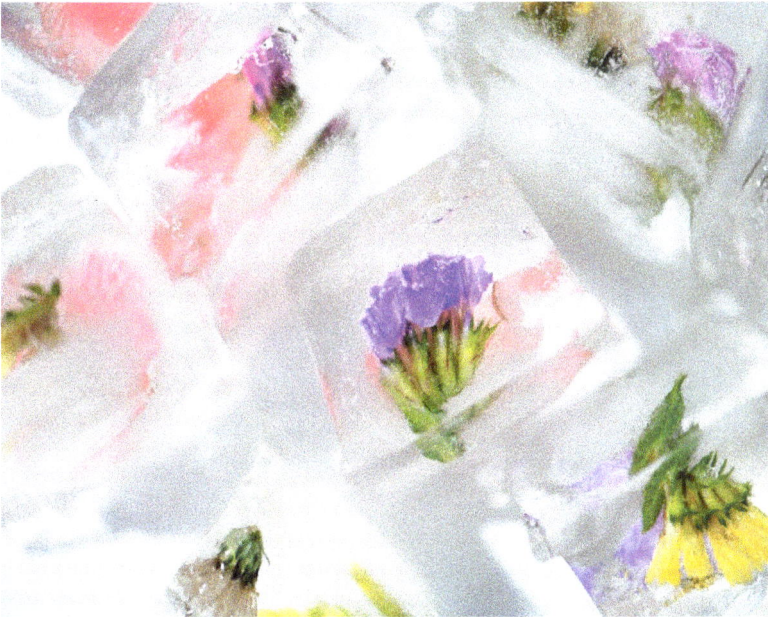

Herbs not included

"Do no harm" - Hippocrates

If you are well educated in the art of herbal teas, when you read this book you may notice the omission of a few herbs and teas you may consider a good choice. There are a few that have been intentionally omitted. This is due to their strong potency and their ability to do harm if not consumed in the correct manner, or if health conditions are not fully assessed before use. Bladderwrack also known as seawrack is one such tea. I would strongly advise that if you are going to use this herb or others not mentioned in this book, you do so under the guidance of a trained professional.

Herbal Synergy

Synergy refers to the combining of substances to achieve a more desirable outcome, in comparison to using them alone. Therefore, we blend tea. For example; choosing a tea that has the potential to assist with hot flushes blended with a tea that has potential to assist with sleep. By doing this you have increased your betterment with just one tea, rather than having to drink multiple different cups.

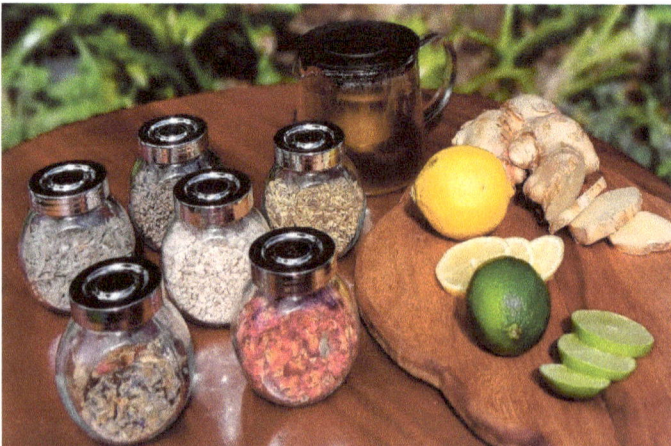

Section 2

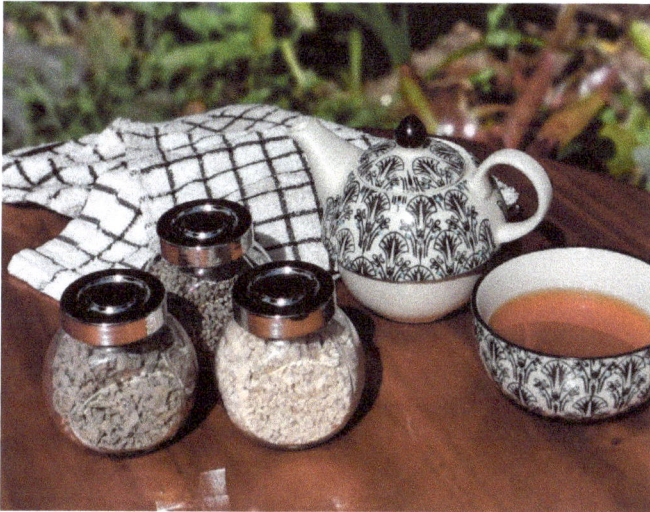

Agrimony

Agrimonia eupatoria

To encourage the reduction of menstrual bleeding or excessive vaginal discharge. This herb is good for people with high blood pressure who are not medicated. Consult your health care professional before using agrimony if you are on medication either allopathic or natural to treat blood pressure.

Agrimony has strong pleasant flavour traditionally used to assist with sleep.

How to brew

Infusion: Dried leaf -Steep 1-2 teaspoons per cup in boiling water for 10-15 minutes.

Fresh leaf- lightly crush 3 teaspoons per cup and steep in boiling water for 10-15 minutes.

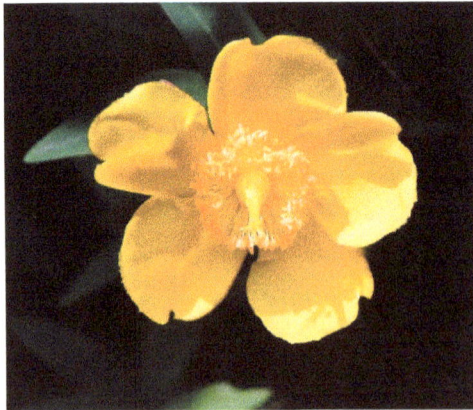

Alfalfa

Medicago sativa

Alfalfa is also known as Lucerne, Lucerne grass and Holy hay. Alfalfa tea plants have deep roots which are able to draw many nourishing nutrients from the soil resulting in alfalfa providing the consumer with vitamin A, D, E and K as well as minerals calcium, phosphorous, potassium and iron.

Drinking alfalfa tea has been shown to assist in the reduction of hot flushes and night sweats. A great blend for this is alfalfa and sage, as sage possesses these attributes also.

For women experiencing hot flushes and night sweats accompanied by joint pain, alfalfa is an excellent choice.

Troubled sleep may be resolved by blending some nettle with your alfalfa for a pre-bed tea.

How to brew

Infusion: Dried leaf -Steep 1-2 teaspoons per cup in boiling water for 10-15 minutes

Fresh leaf- lightly crush 3 teaspoons per cup and steep in boiling water for 10-15 minutes.

Decoction: Use 1 tablespoon of crushed seeds. Boil 2 cups of water add crushed seeds and simmer gently for 5-10 minutes.

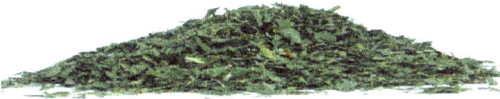

Angelica

Angelica sinensis

Angelica, also known as Dong Quai, means "return to order". The roots are used to make tea. It is thought that the phytosterols, a precursor to sex hormones, and phytoestrones in angelica are the reason it may help reduce hot flushes. This ability to assist with the balancing of hormones aligns it to assisting women suffering from migraines and cramping. It also has a mild calming action that may assist with mood swings, anxiety and irritability. It is also used to treat constipation.

How to brew

Infusion: Dried leaf -Steep 1 teaspoons per cup in boiling water for 10-15 minutes. Fresh leaf- lightly crush 3 teaspoons per cup and steep in boiling water for 10-15 minutes.

Decoction: 1 Tablespoon crushed or ground seeds or 30 gm crushed roots -. Boil 2 cups of water add seeds or roots and simmer gently for 5-10 minutes.

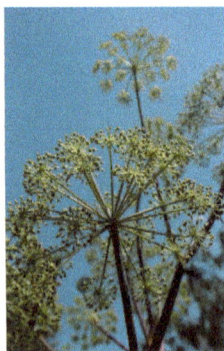

Do not use if you are experiencing heavy menstrual bleeding. Not recommended for pregnant women or children or if using blood thinning medication. Caution should be taken if you have oestrogen sensitive cancer. Angelica contains furocoumarins which increase skin sensitivity to sunlight and may cause dermatitis.

Anise Seeds

Pimpinell anisum

Do not confuse with Star anise (*Illieium verum*) which is covered later in the book.

If you are the kind of women who has trouble putting on weight or suffers from dysmenorrhea, that is painful periods, this may be the tea for you.

Other benefits may be gained from its ability to assist with muscle relaxation and as an anticonvulsant. This is not to be used in place of anticonvulsant medication.

Research has identified anise seeds as having been effective in reducing the frequency and severity of hot flushes.

How to brew

Infusion: Use 1 teaspoons of dried leaf or 3 teaspoons of fresh leaves per cup in boiling water. Steep for 10 minutes

Decoction - crush or grind seeds use 1 tablespoon to 2 cups of water bring to boil and then gently simmer for 5-10 minutes.

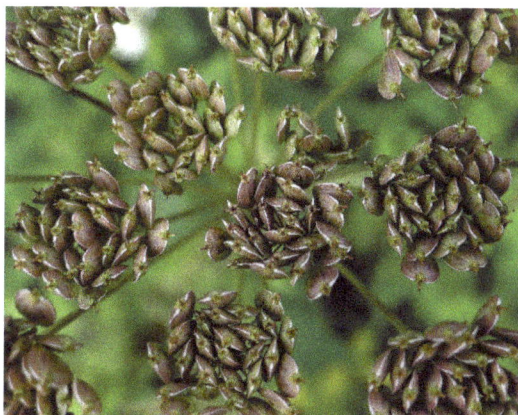

Astragalus

Astragalus membranaceus / mongholicus

When sourcing your own astragalus ensure it is astragalus membranaceus as some varieties are poisonous.

The astragalus root is used for making tea. It is combined with other herbs to assist hot flushes and night sweats, anxiety and depression. Astragalus may assist with weight loss and helps boost the immune system.

Traditionally used in combination with ginseng to address fatigue and candidiasis as well as the herpes simplex virus.

How to brew

Decoction: Use root - add 3-5 grams per cup to your decoration mix and follow instructions for other herbs. (If you are brewing 4 or more cups use the lower amount i.e. 3x4=12 grams.)

Root powder- add to your tea infusion 3 grams a cup.

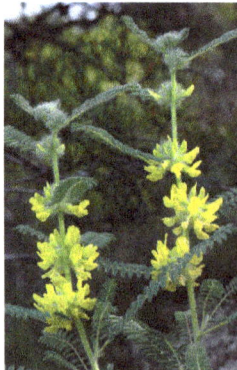

Talk to your health care provider before using astragalus if you are taking lithium or medication to suppress your immune system or if you are using blood thinning medication. Do not use if pregnant or breastfeeding.

Bearberry

Arctostaphylos uva-ursi

Bearberry is used to address the symptoms of urinary tract infections and may be a useful herb to include in your tea blend when experiencing UTIs.

Do not use bearberry for longer than one week and if you are taking any medication please consult your health care provider before use.

How to brew

Infusion: 1 teaspoon of dried leaves per cup of water and let steep for 10-12 hours cover with a cloth. Maximum 2-3 cups daily for 7 days.

Decoction: Place in a saucepan 1 tablespoon of fresh leaves or 1-2 teaspoons of dried leaves in 2 cups of water, bring boil and simmer for 30-40 minutes. Until you are left with one cup of liquid.

Drink half a cup twice daily for a maximum of 7 days.

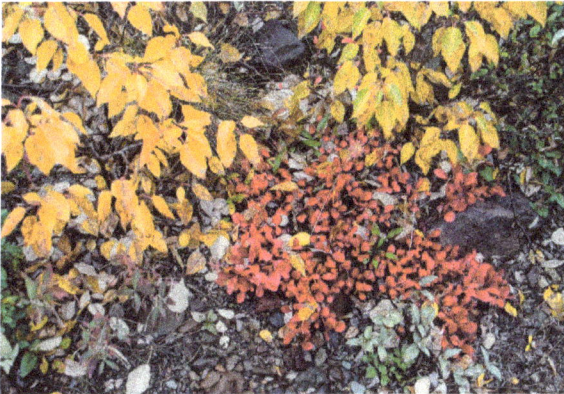

Do not use if pregnant or breastfeeding. Not recommended for children. Do not use if you have kidney or liver issues or taking medication containing lithium.

Betony

Stachy officinalis

Betony is traditionally used to address urinary tract infections, headaches, anxiety and nerve pain.

For menopausal women who are feeling out of sorts, experiencing UTI's and are looking for a bit of a pick-me-up betony may be a good consideration for your tea blend.

Dizziness, low libido and gout may all be assisted by betony.

Combines well with licorice, withania and hawthorn.

How to brew

Infusion: Use1 teaspoon of dried herb. Alternatively, 3 teaspoons of crushed fresh herbs to one cup of boiling water as an infusion.

A little goes a long way with Betony, one cup a day should do the job nicely. Contains tannins do not over consume.

If you are blending with other teas and consuming 3 cups a day, half a teaspoon per cup will be enough.

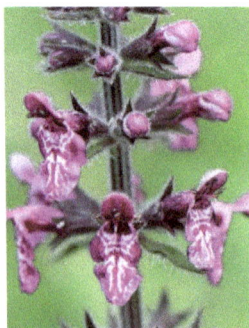

Betony may lower blood pressure and cause diarrhoea, for this reason is not advised during pregnancy. Stop using 2 weeks before surgery.

Borage

Borago officinalis

Borage is a prickly herb that irritates the skin on contact you will need to wear gloves when harvesting fresh product. If you are growing your own gather it in the morning when the dew is still on it to gain the most benefit from its oil components.

Peri-menopausal women may find borage beneficial as it may decrease menstrual cramping, regulate hormones and help with irregular periods.

Feeling stressed? Borage tea may be of assistance.

Borage may induce sweating in some people so it may not be conducive for women plagued with hot flushes and night sweats.

How to brew

Infusion: Use 1 teaspoon of dried leaf or 3 teaspoons of lightly crushed fresh leaves per cup of boiling water. Steep for 10 -15 minutes.

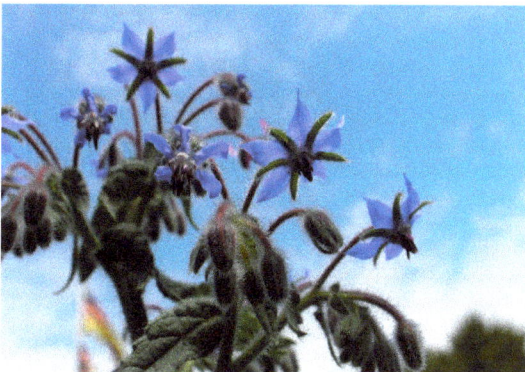

Tea for Menopause

Burnet

Poterium samguisorba

A great tea for women experiencing heavy menstrual blood flow as burnet's astringent properties help to reduce flow.

It is also used to assist with hot flushes and haemorrhoids.

Traditionally used to treat bacterial infections in the urinary tract.

How to brew

Infusion: Use 1 teaspoons of dried leaf or 3 teaspoons of lightly crushed fresh leaf per cup in boiling water. Steep for 10-15 minutes.

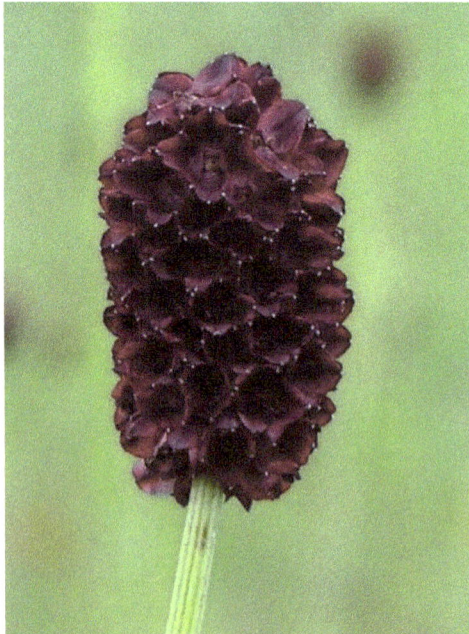

Calendula

Calendula officinalis

Also known as Marigold.

May be of particularly interesting to the peri-menopausal women whose period is all over the place. Calendula is attributed with the potential to modulate menstruation and assist with cramping and other pains associated with menstruation.

Hot flushes add some calendula to your tea blend. Calendula may also assist with digestive disorders.

If you are experiencing vaginal itching and discomfort you can to add some calendula tea to your bath and have a nice relaxing soak.

How to brew

Infusion: Tea can be made of the whole flower or just the petals. The petals are considered less bitter.

Use 2 teaspoons of dried flowers or petals per cup of boiling water or 4 teaspoons of fresh flowers or petals per cup of boiling water. Steep 5-10 minutes.

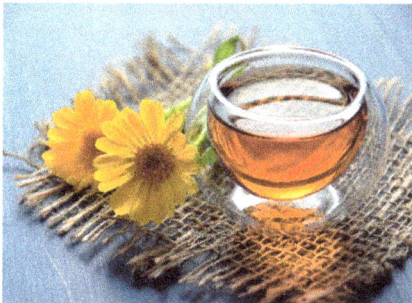

People allergic to chamomile, echinacea and other members of the Asteraceae/compositae family should avoid using calendula. Do not use calendula if pregnant. If you are on medication to treat diabetes, blood pressure or using muscle relaxants without first consulting your health care professional.

Caraway seed

Carum carvi

Caraway seeds are known to assist with digestive complaints. For the women going through the menopausal transition caraway seed tea may reduce weight gain or assist with weight loss when combined with physical activity.

You may ask why to combine with physical activity. Physical activity works in a couple of keyways to assist women in menopause. It gets the body moving with assists with the elimination of waste and hormones. It also helps to reduce fat stores and converts fat to muscle. Knowing your percentage of body fat and muscle before you start an exercise program will help to let you know that even if you aren't losing weight you are swapping fat for muscle which is a good thing.

How to brew

Infusion: 1 teaspoon of caraway seed per cup of boiling water. Steep to taste.

Decoction: 1-2 teaspoons of crushes or ground seed, per cup of water, bring to boil and steep for 10 minutes.

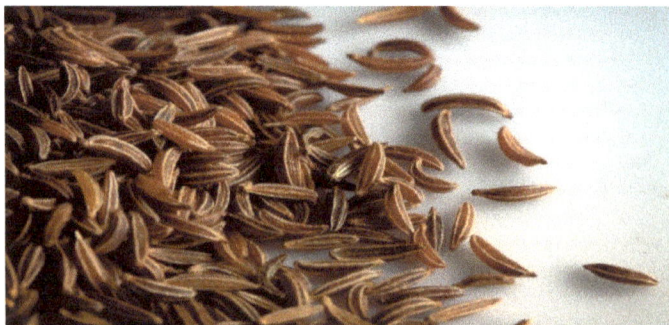

Catnip

Nepeta cataria

Catnip is a member of the mint family and is a fabulous tea to consider if you are feeling anxious, depressed and stressed it contains nepetalactone and inositol constituents accredited with having calming and relaxing effect on people.

It may also assist with menstrual cramping.

If you are retaining fluid the diuretic effect of catnip may be beneficial.

Folic acid is also present in catnip which assists with iron absorption, perfect if you suffer from anaemia.

How to brew

Infusion: Dried leaf -Steep 1-2 teaspoons per cup in boiling water for 5-10 minutes.

Fresh leaf- lightly crush 3 teaspoons per cup in boiling water, steep for 5-10 minutes.

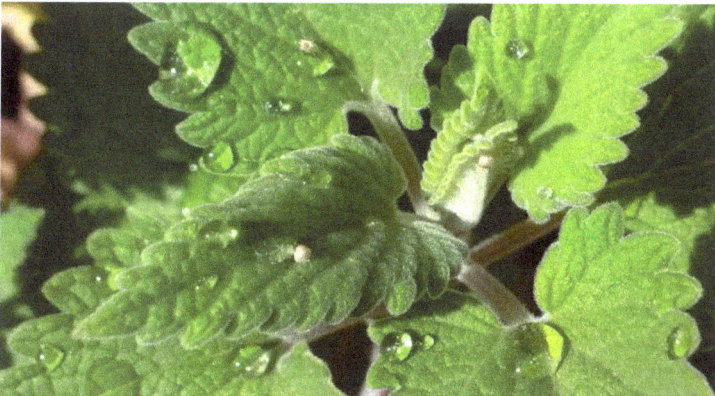

Catuaba Bark

Erythroxylum vaccinifolium

Trichilla catigua

Catuaba comes from two trees in the Amazon rain forest and is used as an aphrodisiac. It is believed that the constituent yohimbine in catuaba bark increases libido for both men and women.

Another constituent of catuaba bark is catuabine which is attributed with stimulating the nervous system thus having the potential to benefit those who are nervous or anxious.

If you're feeling out of sorts, moody, or having issues with your memory then this may be the tea for you.

How to brew

Infusion: 1-2 teaspoons of bark per cup of boiling water. Steep 10-15 minutes.

Decoction: Bark may be added to your decoction mix.

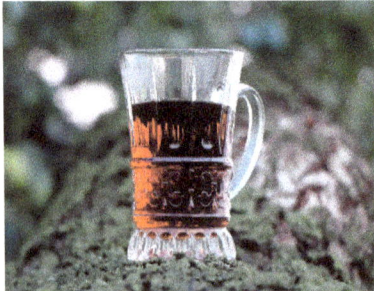

Do not use if pregnant or breast feeding.

Chamomile

Matricaria chamomilla

More than one million cups of chamomile tea are consumed worldwide daily.

Drinking chamomile tea may assist with anxiety and sleep issues.

It has also been shown to assist with decreasing bacteria that cause urinary infections.

Bathing in chamomile tea may also assist with vaginitis a condition some women experience during the menopausal years.

How to brew

Infusion: Dried leaf - 2 teaspoons per cup in boiling water steep for 10-30 minutes.

Fresh leaf- 1 tablespoon per cup of fresh flower and steep in boiling water for 10-30 minutes.

Chamomile tea is also lovely cold.

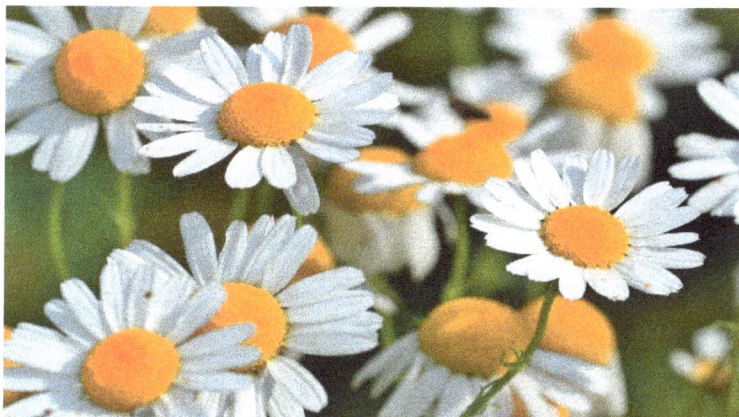

Cinnamon

Cinnamomun verum

Cinnamomum zeylanicum

While cinnamon isn't exactly considered a tea, it is a spice menopausal woman may wish to add to their tea. If you are experiencing higher than normal blood pressure you may find it useful due to its constituent cinnamaldehyde which is believed to assist in the reduction of both systolic and diastolic blood pressure.

Some find cinnamon useful when they are feeling stressed. It also can help to reduce sugar cravings. If using large amounts of cinnamon be aware of the variety you are using. Cassia variety is not recommended in large amounts.

When you make your tea inhale the aroma as you wait for it too steep for added benefit.

How to brew

Infusion: Add ¼ of a teaspoon of cinnamon power to tea blend and stir in allow tea too steep as recommendations for other teas. Bark may be added (grated or whole) to tea and steep for 10-15 minutes.

Decoction: Use a 3-5cm pieces of cinnamon in a decoction, boil as per rest of ingredients, approximately 10-20 minutes.

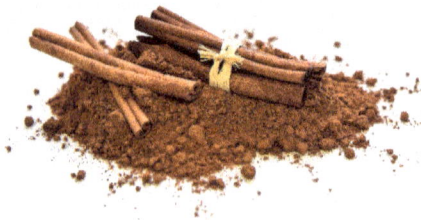

Damiana

Turnera diffusa

Hot flushes, vaginal dryness and irritation. Need a lift to your libido? Then damiana could be the tea for you.

Damiana may assist with mood and anxiety associated with hormone fluctuations in menopause.

It may also assist with regulation of menstruation and headaches associated with menstruation and hormone changes.

How to brew

Infusion: 1-2 teaspoons of dried leaves per cup of boiling water.

Steep 10-20 minutes. Strain and consume.

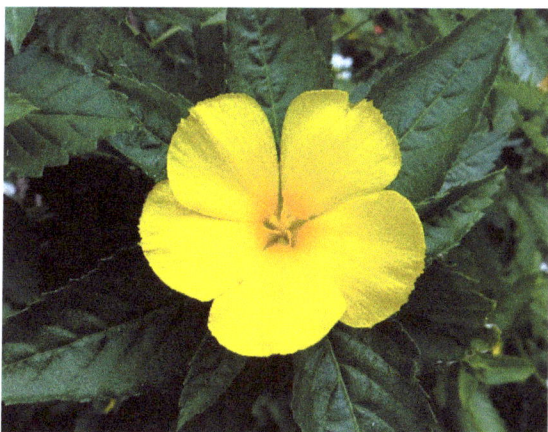

Do not consume if pregnant. Damiana may lower iron absorption, if taking iron supplements take damiana a few hours before or after supplements. Check with your health care professional.

Devils claw

Harpagophytum procumbens

Devils claw is used to address painful inflammation associated with joints such as osteoarthritis and gout.

It may assist with appetite and weight control although the science behind this has not yet been tested.

How to brew

Decoction: Place one teaspoon of chopped and crushed root or root powder in a saucepan with 500mls of cold water. Bring to boil and simmer for 5 minutes. Strain, cool and consume.

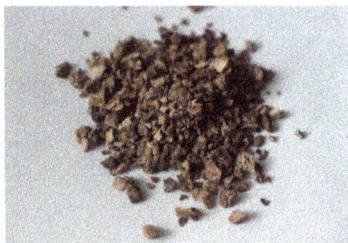

Do not consume if pregnant. Do not use if taking blood thinning medication, it may enhance potency of the medication. If using NSAIDs as it may slow absorption. If using other medication check with your health care provider before using devils claw.

Dill

Antheum graveolens

Dill tea may be made from both the leaves and the seeds of the plant. Both supply a wide range of vitamins and mineral. Seeds are the richer part of the plant and may be beneficial to the peri-menopausal women suffering from painful menses. Dill is phytoestrogenic and as such may assist menopausal women with hot flush, vaginitis and anxiety.

Dill tea is used for assisting with digestive issues such as heartburn and indigestion as it stimulates bile and digestive juices.

It may assist stomach muscles to relax and assist with the removal of gas.

How to brew

Infusion: Use 1-2 teaspoons of crushed seeds or 2-3 teaspoons of fresh leaves per cup of boiling water. Steep for 10-20 minutes. Consume.

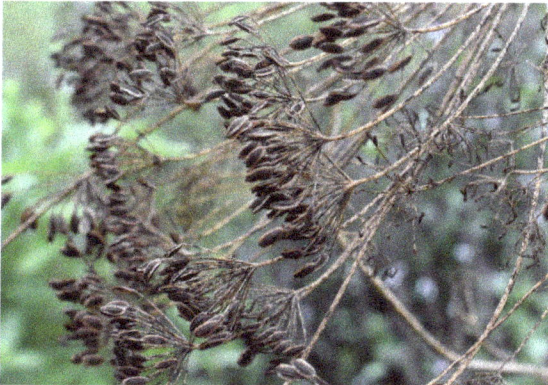

Do not use dill if you are taking lithium without consulting your health care professional. Do not use in pregnancy without consulting your health care professional.

Echinacea

Echinacea purpurea

Echinacea angustifolia

Echinacea has been shown to assist the immune system and in reliving cold and flu symptoms. For the menopausal women echinacea may be of assistance if you are feeling anxious and stressful.

Traditionally used to assist with urinary tract infections, it may be worth a consideration when choosing a tea blend.

How to brew

Leaves, flowers and roots may all be used to make echinacea tea.

Infusion: 1-2 teaspoons of dried herb or 2-4 tablespoon of fresh herb per cup of boiling water. Steep for 10-15 minutes. Strain and consume.

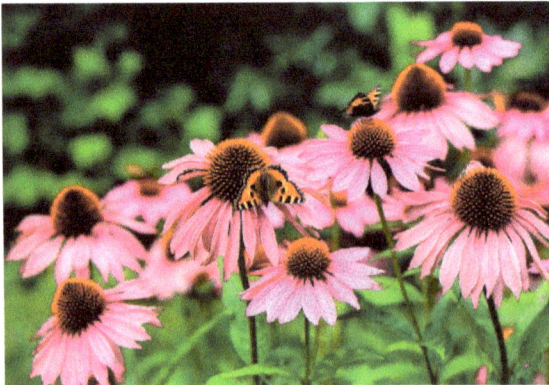

Do not use echinacea if you have an auto immune condition without discussing it with your health care professional. Not recommended for children under two.

Evening Primrose

Oenothera biennis

Evening primrose has the potential to reduce the severity of hot flushes. Unfortunately, it does not appear to reduce the frequency therefore it would be recommended that it was used with other herbs to produce a synergistic effect.

Many people use evening primrose oil to address menopause symptoms this is because of the high concentrations of Gamma-linolenic acid (GLA) found in evening primrose. While most studies are done on the oil, the tea may be beneficial to women suffering from hot flushes, breast pain, as well as irritability and bloating.

The root of the evening primrose is traditionally used in tea to treat obesity. Leaves and roots are drunk as a tea to relieve an upset stomach.

How to brew

Infusion: Fresh flowers or leaves 1-2 teaspoon per cup of boiling water, steep for 3-5 minutes.

Decoction: Add a 5cm piece of evening primrose crushed fresh root or 2-3 teaspoon of dried root to your decoction simmer for 10-15 minutes, cool and consume.

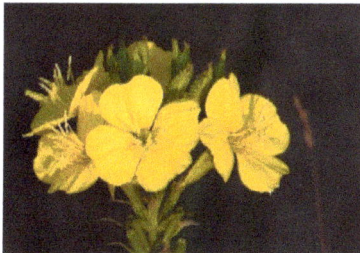

People with epilepsy should consult their health care professional before using this tea. Do not use if pregnant.

Fennel

Foeniculum vulgare

Fennel may assist menopausal women having problems sleeping, including those experiencing night sweats.

If you are feeling moody, anxious or having memory issues add some fennel to your tea mix.

Phytoestrogenic properties of fennel are thought to be the reason it may assist with vaginal dryness for menopausal women.

Fennel has also been found to be of great assistance for menstrual pain.

How to brew

Infusion: Uses leaves. 3 teaspoons of fresh leaves or 2 teaspoons of dried leaves per cup of boiling water. Steep to taste.

Decoction: Uses seeds. 1 tablespoon of crushed seed to 2 cups of boiling water, simmer gently 5 to 10 minutes.

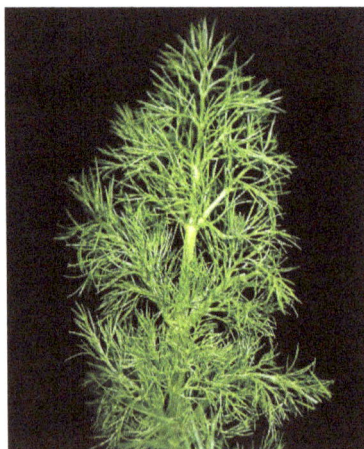

Fenugreek

Trigonella foenum-graccum

Fenugreek seeds have been shown to decrease the frequency of hot flushes and night sweats. Fenugreek is a highly nourishing plant the leaves contain calcium, zinc, and iron as well as good amounts of vitamin C.

Fenugreek may also assist with inflammation associated with rheumatoid arthritis, a condition which is associated with hormone fluctuations that can occur during menopause.

Fenugreek tea made from the seeds is a great tea to consider if you are diabetic due to its ability to lower blood sugars. The seeds also contain fibre which assist with constipation.

How to brew

Infusion: Use 1 teaspoon of dried leaves or 3 teaspoons of fresh leaves per cup of boiling water and steep. Is particularly good with alfalfa.

Decoction: Use one teaspoon per cup of water, boil until seeds are soft, for higher nutritional value leave the seeds in your tea and consume them.

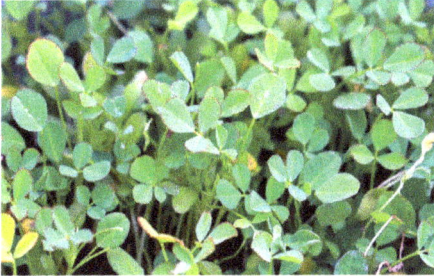

Do not consume if pregnant as it may induce labour. People with peanut allergies may also be allergic to fenugreek.

Flaxseed/Linseed

Linum usitatissimum

Flaxseed tea contains lignans which are thought to play a role in why flaxseed appears to assist with the reduction of hot flushes and night sweats. Flaxseed is a great source of fibre which assists with hormone clearance and prevention of constipation.

Some have found flaxseed helps to negate sleep issues associated with menopause.

How to brew

Infusion: Use 1 teaspoon of ground flaxseed or 2 teaspoon of meal per cup of boiling water. Steep 10-15 minutes. Strain if desired.

Cinnamon is often used as an accomplishment with flaxseed tea.

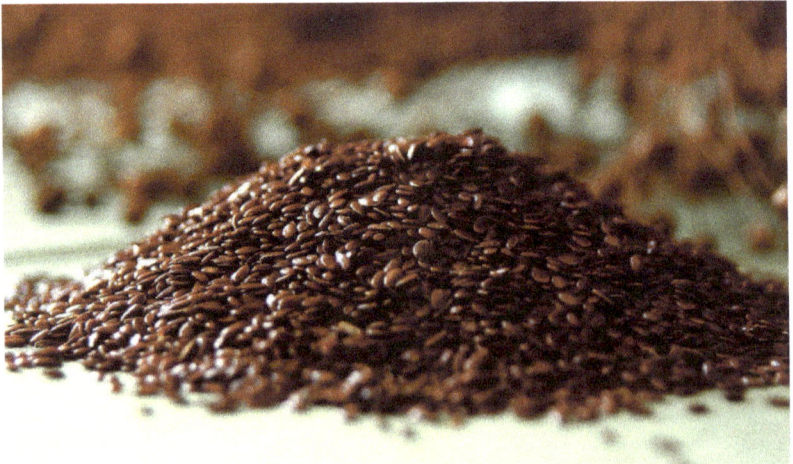

Geranium

Geranium robertiamum, Geranium pelargonium odoratissimum

WARNING not all geraniums are edible please double check the botanical name of your geranium to ensure it is edible and if in doubt do not use in your tea.

Geranium can be of assistance with high blood pressure and migraines. The leaves of geranium have a mild endorphin release effect thus may assist with pain and reduce stress.

Tea from the flowers of *Geranium robertiamum* has been shown to assist with headaches and bloating. While a decoction of the leaves and roots may assist with cholesterol levels.

How to brew

Infusion: Flowers or leaves, 1 teaspoon of dried or 3 teaspoons fresh crushed leaves per cup of boiling water. Steep for 10-15 minutes.

Decoction: 2-3 teaspoons of root or leaves. Roots go in with cold water as bring to boil, then simmer. Add leaves to simmering water, simmer both for 10-15 minutes.

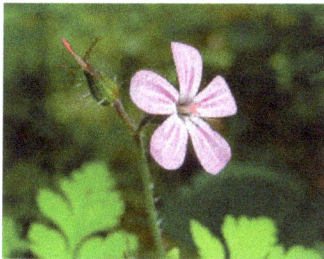

Do not consume if pregnant or lactating.

Ginger

Zingiber officinale

What a little powerhouse a piece of ginger is!

Full disclosure, ginger is my absolute favourite flavour and I add it to almost anything.

For the menopausal woman you will find ginger is regularly used to assist with hot flushes and night sweats, to assist with joint pain and osteoporosis, nausea and menstrual cramps, bloating and digestive disorders.

How to brew

Infusion on own or with other herbs.10cm piece of ginger peeled and chopped or grated, added to 1 cup of boiling water and steep for 10-15 minutes.

Decoction on own or with other herbs.10 cm piece of ginger peeled, chopped or grated. I personally don't peel my ginger, but it may depend where you source it from, if it is organic just give it a good wash. Add 300 ml of water and slowly bring to boil, simmer for 5 minutes with lid on. May be drank hot or cold.

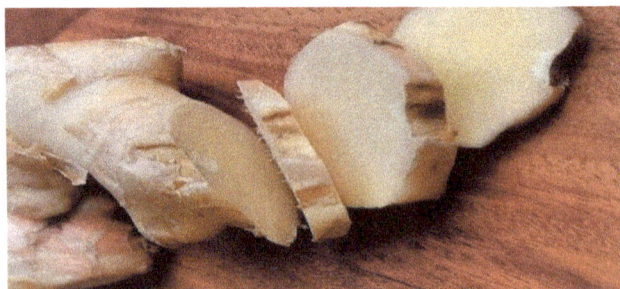

Do not use ginger if on medication for gallstones or blood thinning medication without clearance for your health care professional.

Ginseng - American

Panax quinquefolius

Ginseng - Korean

Panax ginseng

Please note these are two of three ginseng varieties mentioned in this book. Refer to the botanical name when sourcing.

Both ginsengs may assist with cognitive function, memory loss, anxiety, stress and fatigue. Both the American and Korean ginseng are traditionally used to assist with sleep, nerve pain and headaches.

Studies are limited on exactly how ginseng assists women with menopause; however, many women swear by it.

How to brew

Infusion: Grate or grind dried ginseng root. Add 1-2 tablespoons per cup of off the boil water and steep for 5-10 minutes. Strain and consume.

Dried root may also be used in a decoction just add it once the water has finished boiling if using other herbs as boiling water may destroy beneficial elements. Steep for 15-20 minutes.

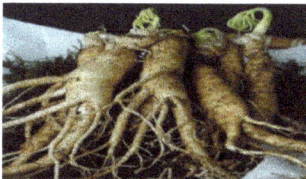

Do not take if pregnant. May lower blood pressure and blood sugar seek assistance from your health care professional if in doubt of interaction with medication. Stop 2 weeks before surgery.

Ginseng - Siberian

Eleutherococcus senticosus

Siberian ginseng has adaptogenic properties which may help you to cope with the pressures of daily life and reduce stress. It may also assist with fatigue and sleep issues, including insomnia.

For the menopausal woman it may assist with reducing weight gain, hot flushes, and irritability. It is also used to improve libido.

How to brew

Infusion: Grate or shave 1 tablespoon worth of ginseng root into a tea ball. Boil water and pour into cup, add tea ball to cup. Steep for 5 -10 minutes. Consume.

Ginseng may also be added to your decoction mix.

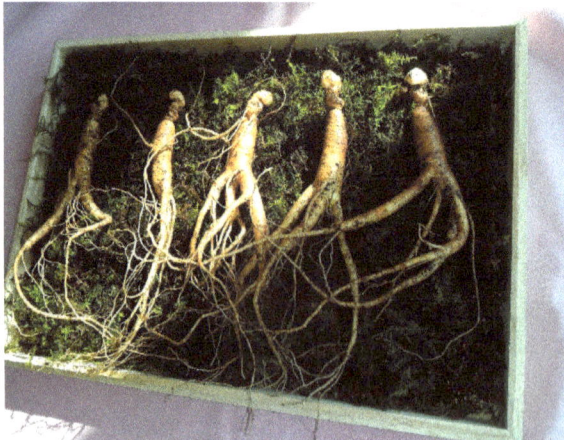

If taking medication for depression including lithium, check with your health care provider before using ginseng. If you have a bleeding disorder, heart condition or hormone sensitive condition check with your health care professional before us.

Goldenrod

Solidago virgaurea. Solidago canadensis and Solidago odora

While goldenrod isn't specifically indicated to treat menopause, it has the potential to assist with conditions that go along with the menopausal transition including urinary tract infections and dysuria.

This is an herb you may consider putting in an herbal blend.

How to brew

Infusion: 1 heaped teaspoon of dried herb or 3 teaspoons of fresh young leaves and flowers in one cup of boiling water. Steep for 10 minutes. Strain and drink.

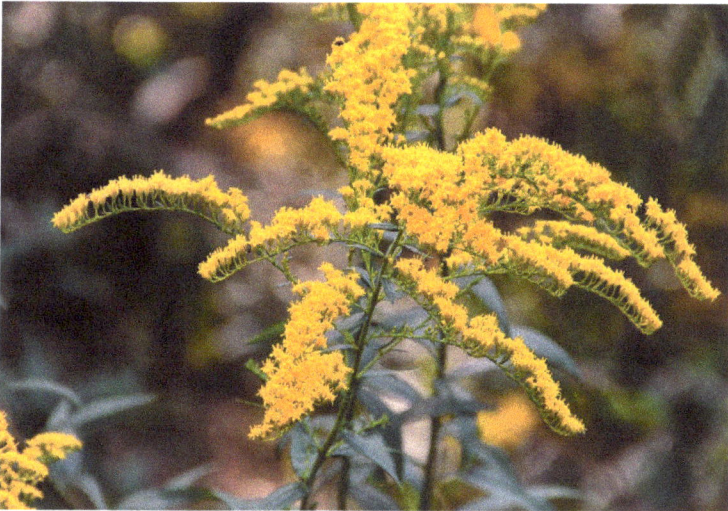

Do not use if taking a diuretic for high blood pressure, if unsure if you are taking one check with your prescribing physician before using goldenrod.

Gotu kola

Centella asiatica

Gotu kola is regarded as having the properties with the potential to increase cognition due to a protein that appears to increase the growth reach of dendrites. This may be of benefit to women who are experiencing cognitive decline as they transition through menopause. It has the potential to improve mood.

The anti-inflammatory properties of gout kola may also assist women who are experiencing joint pain. Gotu kola may also assist with reducing hair loss and anxiety. It may also assist with panic attacks.

Gotu kola is a diuretic and may be used to assist urinary tract infections. An added benefit of Gotu kola is its ability to inhibit enzymes that break down collagen. What woman wouldn't love that!

How to brew

Infusion: 1 teaspoon of dried herb or 2-3 teaspoons of fresh leaves and stem in one cup of boiling water. Steep for 10 minutes. Strain and drink.

Do not drink more than 3 cups a day. Recommended for short term use.

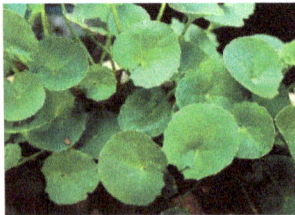

Gotu kola can increase the effects of some medications including ibuprofen and ketamine. Check with your health care professional before using Gotu kola if you are taking medications. May increase photosensitivity. Do not use in pregnancy.

Hawthorne

Crataegus pinnatifida

If you are worried about cardiovascular health as you go through menopause then hawthorn may be the herb for you. Hawthorne has been shown to lower diastolic heart rate and may assist with erratic heart beats and palpitations.

How to brew

Infusion: Use 1 teaspoon of dried leaves and/or flowers or 3 teaspoons of fresh leaves and/or flowers per cup of boiling water. Steep 5-10 minutes. Strain and consume.

Decoction: Use 1 tablespoon of dried berries in 2 cups of boiling water, simmer for 10-15 minutes with lid on.

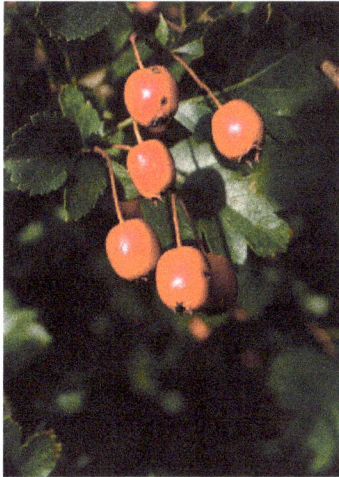

Do not use Hawthorne if you are taking medication to lower your blood pressure or taking heart medication please check with your prescribing physician before using Hawthorne. Stop use 2 weeks prior to surgery.

Heather

Calluna vulgaris

Heather can help remove toxins from your body, so it is great it you are suffering from gout. It has been traditionally used to treat rheumatism and arthritis.

Assisting sleep is also another area where heather may be of benefit. Heather tea is often used to assist with bladder infections and is recommended as a short-term tea when symptoms are occurring.

How to brew

Infusion: Use both flowers and leaves. Place 2 heaped teaspoons in 1 cup of boiling water, steep for 10-15 minutes. Consume.

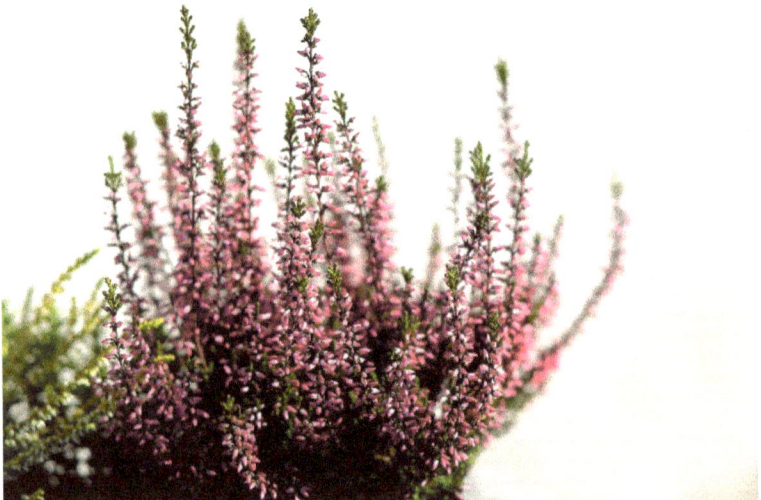

There is some thought that long term therapeutic use of heather may not be good for the liver. Seek professional advice before consuming on a regular basis.

Hollyhock

Alcea rosea

The science behind how Hollyhock works is limited, meaning not many studies have been done.

It has been shown to have antimicrobial and anti-inflammatory properties as well as analgesic, antiurolithiatic and immunomodulatory potential.

All parts of the plant can be consumed, the flowers are used for pain relief.

Menopausal women experiencing urinary discomfort and pain hollyhock would be worth considering.

How to brew

Infusion: Fresh flowers, use one handful (3-4 flower heads) of fresh flowers per cup, cover with boiling water and steep for 10-15 minutes. Strain and consume.

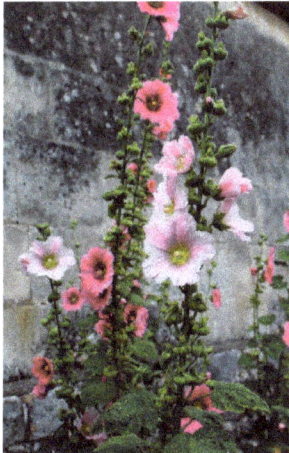

Holy Basil

Ocimum tenuiflorum

Also known as Tulsi. Tulsi has been linked to reduction of cortisol. High stress levels elevate cortisol which can impact on memory and weight gain.

Traditionally used for migraines and headaches as well as for arthritis.

How to brew

Infusion: 1 teaspoon of dried herb or 3 teaspoons of fresh herb per cup of hot water. If you leave the fresh herb to wilt for 24 hours you will get a stronger flavour. Steep 10-15 minutes. May be consumed hot or cold. May be used to make iced tea.

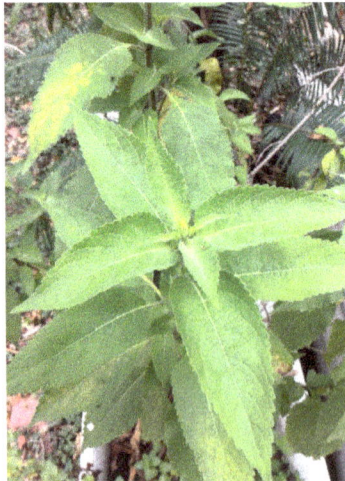

Do not consume large amounts if trying to fall pregnant or if pregnant. May lower blood sugar levels, effect blood clotting ability, and lower thyroxine level. If you have any of these issues check with your health care provider before use. Stop use 2 weeks prior to surgery.

Hops

Humlus lupulus

Hops tea may be of benefit to women having hot flushes and night sweats. It also has a sedative element which may assist with sleep quality. Hops may also assist menopausal women suffering from vaginal dryness, itching and discomfort and urinary tract infections.

If you are experiencing anxiety, stress and tight muscles then hops may be of use to you. Hops has a strong taste and combines nicely with chamomile, mint or passionflower.

How to brew

Infusion: 1 teaspoon of dried leaf or 3 teaspoons of freshly crushed leaves per cup of boiling water. Steep to taste.

Decoction: 1 heaped tablespoon of hops flowers (cones) per cup of cold water in a saucepan bring to a simmer for 2-3 minutes, take off heat and steep for 10-15 minutes. Consume.

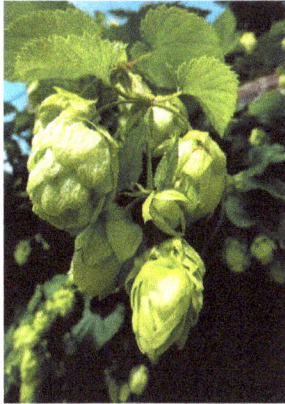

Hops has phytoestrogenic properties so should not be used if you have an estrogen cancer. If you are taking medication for depression or are taking medication that is sedative in nature, please consult a health professional before using hops. Do not use if pregnant or breast feeding and is not recommend for children.

Horsetail

Equisetum arvense

Unfortunately for some women menopause sees them suffering with urinary incontinence. The silica content in horsetail is fabulous for connective tissue that strengthens the pelvic region, which may assist with urinary incontinence. Silica also assists with hair, nail and skin health.

Horsetail may also assist with the treatment of UTI's.

It may also be of assistance if you are suffering from menstrual cramping.

How to brew

Infusion: 2-3 teaspoons of horsetail per cup of boiling water, steep 5-10 minutes.

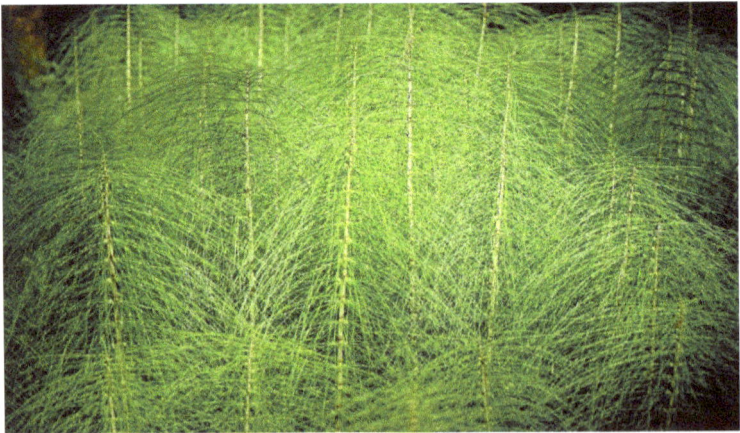

Long-term use of horsetail is not recommended, Horsetail depletes thiamine and potassium. Diabetes please note Horsetail also lowers blood sugars. Do not use if pregnant.

Hydrangea

Hydrangea arborescens

Also known as seven bark herb, due to the seven colours in the root exposed as you peel each layer away. The root of the plant was traditionally used to treat urinary infections and is also thought to help hay fever.

How to brew

The root is harvested in the autumn and dried, then stored in cardboard box or paper bag, storage in plastic may result in mold growth.

Infusion: 1 teaspoon of dried root per cup of boiling water. Steep 3-5 minutes, strain and consume.

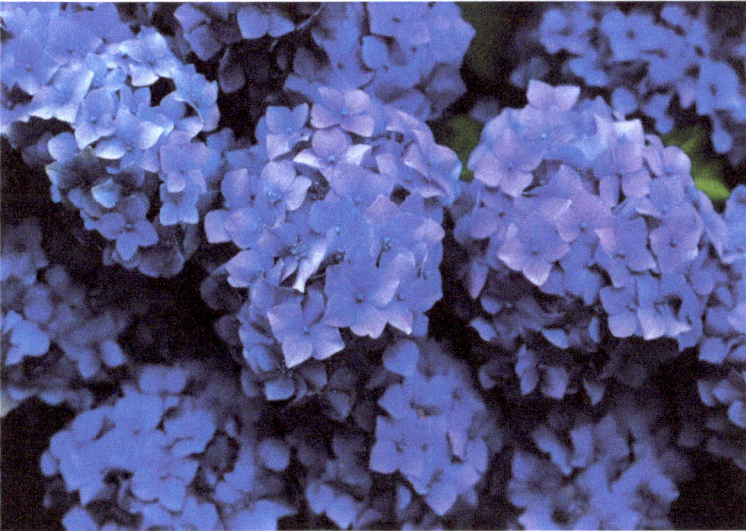

Do not use if you are taking lithium medication as hydrangea may decrease the effectiveness of this medication. Do not use in pregnancy or if breastfeeding.

Hyssop

Hyssopus officinalis

If you are a menopausal woman suffering from digestive issues, including being bloated and gassy. Hyssop is the tea to add to your blend.

It may also help relieve menstrual cramping.

Hyssop has a mild laxative action so keep this in mind when considering adding hyssop to a blend.

Urinary tract infections may also benefit from the use of hyssop.

How to brew

Infusion: Use 1 teaspoons of fresh or dried tops or leaves in one cup of water, steep for 10-30 minutes.

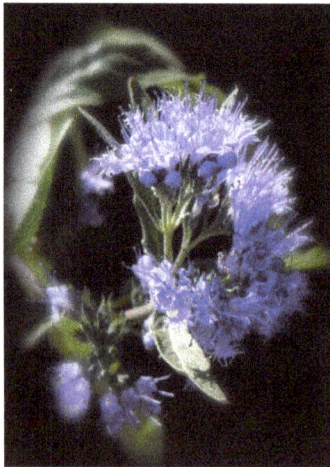

Do not use if pregnant as it may cause bleeding and lead to miscarriage. If you have a history of seizures do not use hyssop without consulting your health care professional.

Jasmine

Jasminum officinale

Jasminum sambac

Commercial jasmine tea is a combination of green tea and the blossom of the jasmine plant. If you are buying pre-blended jasmine tea you are getting the benefits of both green tea and the jasmine. This blend has the potential to assist with weight reduction and fat accumulation.

Feeling moody? Make yourself a cup of jasmine tea and inhale the aroma while it steeps to address autonomic nerve activity and improve your mood.

Jasmine tea may assist with blood sugar regulation and therefore assist women with chocolate cravings, something many menopausal women experience.

How to brew

Infusion: 1 teaspoon of dried flowers or 3 teaspoons of fresh flowers per cup of boiling water. Steep 5-10 minutes.

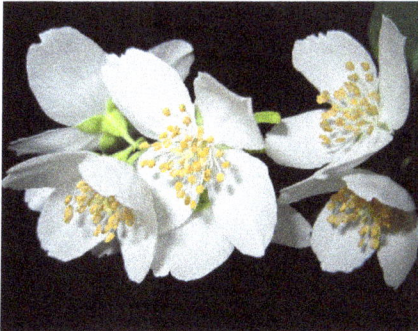

If using commercial jasmine tea, remember green tea has caffeine in it, so it may not be the best tea before bed if you are experiencing sleep issues.

Kava

Piper methysticum

Kava is used to address sleep issues and to improve mood. The rhizome (root) of the plant contains constituents called kavalactones which have extremely effective relaxative properties. You should not operate a car or machinery after having kava.

There are many medications which kava interacts with so please consult with a health care professional before using Kava if you are on medication.

How to brew

Infusion: Use 2-4 tablespoons of Kava powder per cup of hot water from the tap, blend in a blender or with a stick blender, and strain using a fine sieve, cheesecloth or muslin bag. Discard the pulp and drink the liquid.

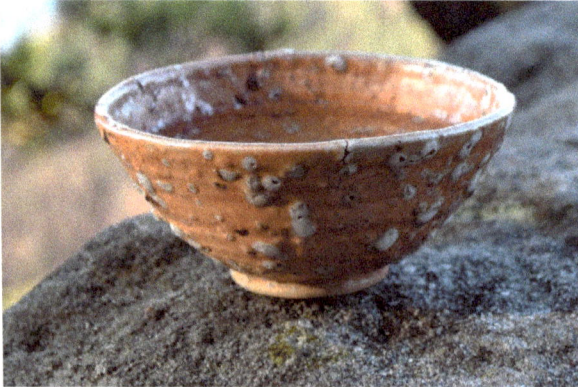

Do not use if pregnant or lactating. If using any medication check with your health care professional before using kava.

Kelp

Saccharina japonica

Also known as Kombu Cha.

Kelp is a wonderful source of iodine as well as calcium, magnesium and sodium which are all great for thyroid health.

For the menopausal woman experiencing changes in hormone levels it is important to monitor your thyroid health. Too much iodine can be just as detrimental to your health as too little, so please see your health care professional before using kelp in therapeutic amounts.

Kelp is considered a blood purifier, which means it helps clear toxins from the body, it is useful if you have arthritis.

How to brew

Infusion:

Option 1. Use ½ -1 teaspoon of kelp powder/tea per cup of boiling water. Do not consume more than 2 teaspoons a day.

Option 2. Use 15 gm of fresh kelp per cup and add hot water. Salt is often added to taste.

The Japanese add plum to the tea to give it a more acidic flavour which gives the tea a pink appearance.

Before using kelp tea for treating menopause it would be advisable to get your iodine levels measured and repeat that test regularly if using kelp tea. Do not use if you have hyperthyroidism are on thyroid medications without the consent of your health care professional.

Tea for Menopause
Kelp Saccharina japonica

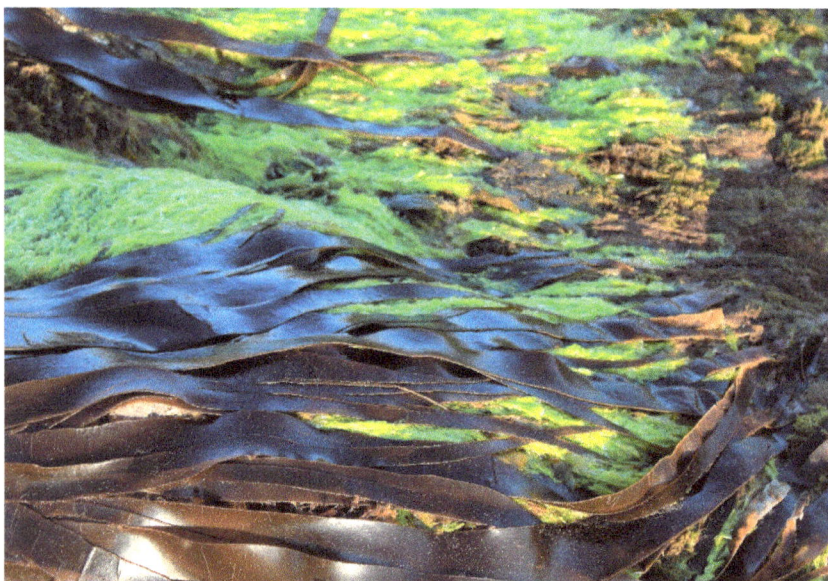

Lavender

Lavandula angustifolia

Inhaling the scent of lavender has been shown to reduce hot flushing so when making lavender tea, inhale ladies, inhale. Drinking lavender tea may assist as it has constituents that possess oestrogenic properties. These may assist with the reduction of hot flushes and night sweats. Lavender is of course accredited with assisting with sleep and stress.

How to brew

Infusion: 1 teaspoon of dried flowers or 3 teaspoons of fresh flowers per cup of boiling water. Steep 5-10 minutes

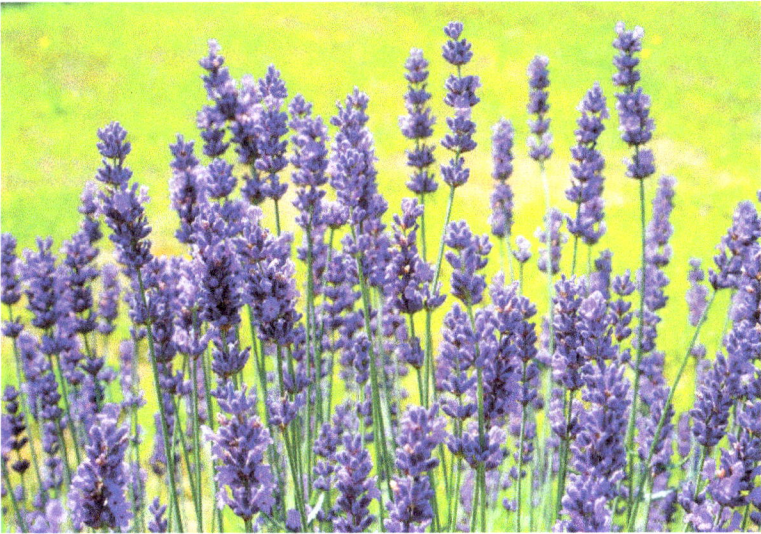

Lemon & Lime

Citrus limon & citrus aurantifolia

How could anyone write a book about tea and not mention the humble citrus, the lemon and the lime. Lemon and lime are added to tea to enhance the taste. There are however many health benefits when you include these to your blend;

Both may increase the antioxidant absorption gained from drinking your tea.

Catechins assist the body to fight disease and boost immunity. The most common one in tea is epigallocatechin gallate often shortened to EGCG. Catechins like an acid environment by adding the lemon or lime to the tea provides the acidity required enhancing the effective uptake of catechins.

Green tea has the most EGCG, however most teas made for Camellia sinensis have catechins. The more fermented the tea is the less EGCG it will have. Sage also contains catechins, so adding lemon or lime to sage tea you increase its potential benefits. Catechins are attributed with stimulating metabolism, reducing body fat and contributing to weight loss.

How to brew

Fresh slices or juice may be added to the finished tea. Dried peel may be added to an infusion or decoction. ½ to 1 teaspoon per cup of water, to achieve desired taste.

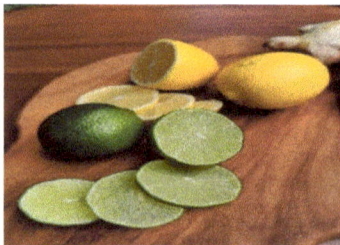

Lemon balm

Melissa officinalis

Lemon balm tea has the potential to reduce anxiety, depression and improve sleep quality.

Lemon balm contains rosmarinic acid which has been shown in animal studies to protect against memory impairments.

Lemon balm may also help with constipation.

Lemon balm may be of assistance for people with overactive thyroids. If you have a thyroid issue check caution below.

How to brew

Infusion: Use 1-2 teaspoons of dried herb per cup of boiling water or 3 teaspoons chopped or crushed fresh leaves per cup of boiling water, steep 10-15 minutes.

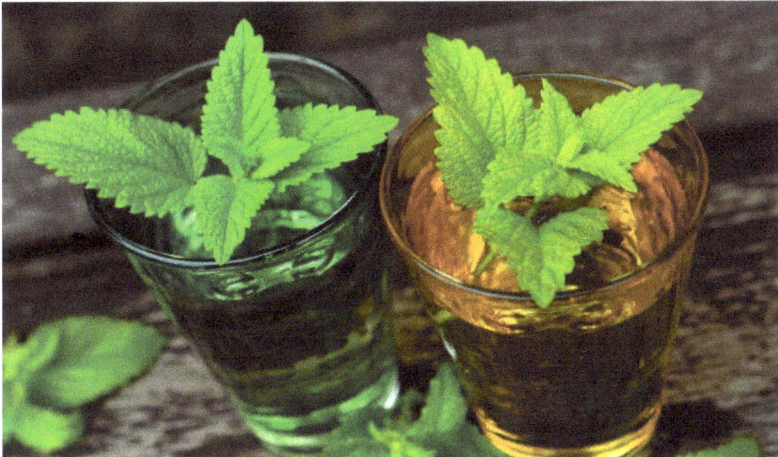

If you are taking medication for hypothyroidism do not use lemon balm, if you are taking medication for hyperthyroidism please consult with your health care professional before using lemon balm.

Lemongrass

Cymbopogon citratus

Lemongrass is a pleasant tasting tea often included in menopausal blends. There are very few studies on lemongrass tea. Traditionally it is used to assist with hot flushes, cramping, digestion, constipation and indigestion.

Many people find lemongrass helps them feel less stressed. It has good levels of potassium which are attributed to its potential to reduce high blood pressure. Lemongrass may also assist in weight loss and lowering cholesterol.

How to brew

Infusion: Use 2-3 leaves chopped add 1 cup boiling water steep 15 minutes.

Decoction: boil 2 cups of water add a 5 cm piece of stalk or 2-3 leaves chopped into 2 cm pieces, boil for 5 minutes strain and consume hot or cold.

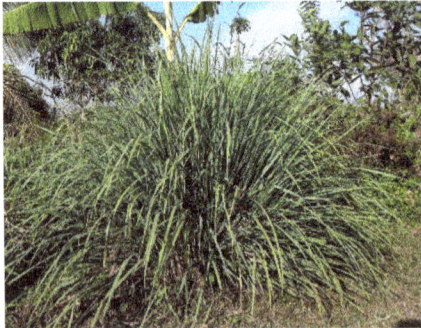

Lemongrass in an emmenagogue which means it may bring on a period, so if you are experiencing heavy bleeding this may not be the herb for you. Do not use if pregnant or breast feeding. Diabetics should consult a health care professional before use as lemongrass may lower sugar levels.

Lemon verbena

Aloysia triphylla, Aloysia citriodora

Lippia citriodora

Lemon verbena may assist those who are bloated and gassy. May be of benefit if you are experiencing digestive issues.

Add it to your night-time tea blend to assist with sleep or use it in your joint pain blend.

Some people like to use lemon verbena to assist with weight loss. With a strong lemon-lime flavour you may choose to add include it in your tea blend.

How to brew

Infusion: 1 teaspoon of dried leaves and flowers, or 3 teaspoons of fresh leaves and flowers per cup of boiling water. Steep covered for 15 minutes. Drink hot or as iced tea.

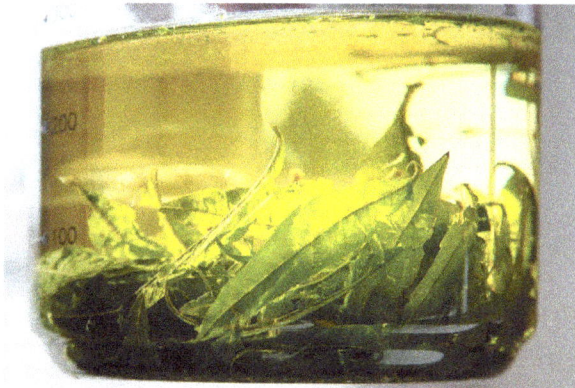

May cause skin irritation is some people, not enough evidence to approve safety in pregnancy or breast feeding so best to avoid.

Licorice

Glycyrrhiza glabra, Glycyrrhiza uralensis, Glycyrrhiza inflata

When suffering from hot flushes and night sweats, licorice is worth considering. If you have low blood pressure and feel dizzy give licorice a try.

Licorice may assist menopausal women with mood swings, anxiety, stress and depression as well as stomach bloating and digestive issues.

Cramping and painful periods may be relieved by the addition of licorice to your tea blend.

How to brew

Infusion or Decoction: 1 teaspoon of crushed or powdered licorice root per cup of water. Steep to taste. Licorice adds a sweet flavour to tea blends and may be drunk hot or cold.

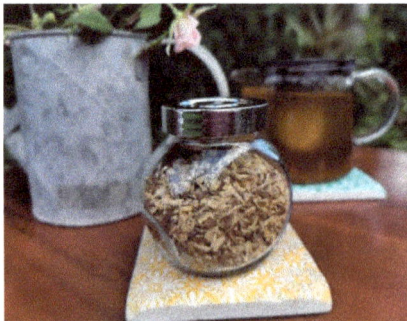

Warfarin: If you are taking warfarin do not use licorice as it may decrease the effectiveness of warfarin. If you are using blood pressure medication, estrogen medication, digoxin or furosemide or other medication to address potassium levels or for kidney or liver please check with your health care provider before using licorice.

Linden

Tilia europaea, Tilia americana,
Tilia Mexicana, Tilia ssp.

From the linden tree, leaves and flowers are used fresh or dried to make tea. The linden tea is an anxiolytic which means it has the potential to reduce anxiety and stress and may be used to assist sleep.

Linden has traditionally been used to assist with headache and migraines, rapid heartbeat, high blood pressure and urinary incontinence.

How to brew

Infusion: 1 teaspoon of dried flowers or leaves per cup of boiling water or 3 teaspoons of fresh flowers or leaves per cup of boiling water. Steep 10-15 minutes.

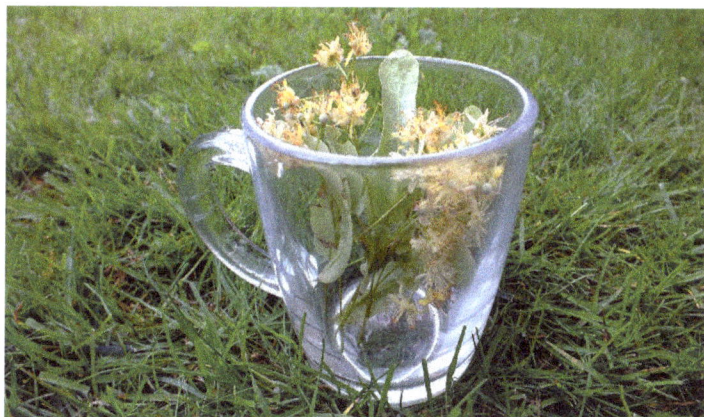

If you are on blood pressure medication, have a history of heart disease or taking lithium, check with your health care professional before using linden. Do not use if pregnant.

Lovage

Levisticum officinale

The quercetin in lovage may be of assistance to people suffering with allergies. For the menopausal woman who is feeling moody, anxious, bloated or suffering from headaches and migraines lovage may be a beneficial herb to add to your tea blend. Lovage is used to bring on menstruation so if you are bleeding frequently or heavily this may not be the tea for you.

Lovage is also used to assist urination and urinary tract infections. Lovage is also indicated for relief from joint pain and gout.

How to brew

Infusion: Use 1 teaspoon of dried lovage leaves or 2 teaspoons of fresh chopped leaves per cup of boiling water. Steep 10-15 minutes. May be consumed hot or cold.

Decoction: Use 1 tablespoon of fruit or grated root in 2 cups of cold water. Bring to boil, reduce heat, simmer until liquid has halved in amount, strain and consume liquid. Drink one third of a cup three times a day.

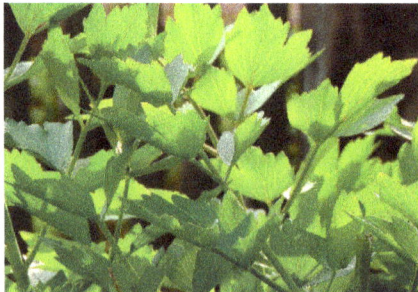

Do not use if you have kidney issues or are taking diuretic drugs. Lovage my induce photosensitivity in some people, thus it is recommended you start a low consumption and increase if no reaction is experienced. Do not use if pregnant.

Marjoram

Origanum majorana

Marjoram would be an herb to consider if you are a sufferer from polycystic ovary syndrome (PCOS). Research has identified that marjoram reduces dehydroepiandrosterone (DHEA) which is often elevated in women with PCOS. Going through menopause does not stop PCOS so a tea with marjoram may benefit the PCOS menopausal woman.

Marjoram may also assist with anxiety and digestive issues.

How to brew

Infusion: 1 teaspoon of dried herb or 2 teaspoons of fresh herb per cup of boiling water. Steep to taste.

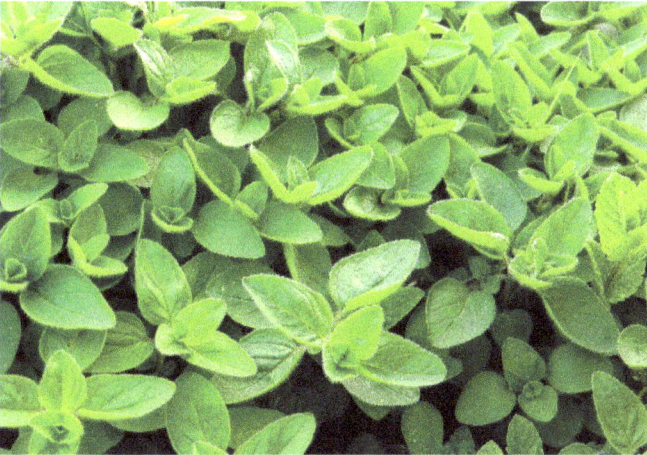

Marjoram interacts with lithium by decreasing lithium excretion. Consult your health care professional before using marjoram if you are taking lithium. Do not use in pregnancy due to its ability to impact on hormone levels. Not enough is known about its safety in breastfeeding.

Marshmallow

Althaea officinalis

Not to be confused with the fluffy sugary sweet.

Marshmallow is a mucilage, which means it helps to treat constipation and assists with the removal of excessive hormones. Marshmallow has the potential to heal mucosal lining throughout the body. These attributes may be of assistance for menopausal women with digestive and absorption issues. Marshmallow tea is a great herb on its own or to add to your urinary or bladder infection blend.

How to brew

Infusion:

Option 1. Fill a glass jar a ¼ full of marshmallow root, fill the jar with boiling water put the lid on the jar. Let steep for 20 minutes, strain and consume.

Option 2. Fill a glass jar a 1/4 full of marshmallow root Use cold filtered water, let steep for 4-12 hours Strain and consume or store in refrigerator and drink over next few days.

Decoction: Use 1 tablespoon of cut marshmallow root per 1.5 cups of cold water. Place water and marshmallow root in a saucepan and bring to boil cover and simmer on low for 20 minutes. Remove from heat and strain through sieve, muslin or cheese cloth. Enjoy.

Seek advice from your health care professional if you are taking lithium or diabetes related drugs before using marshmallow. Avoid if pregnant or breastfeeding. Cease using 2 weeks before surgery. Marshmallow may reduce the absorbency of medication therefore take at least an hour before or after medication. Check with your health professional if you are taking multiple medications before use.

Marshmallow *Althaea officinalis*

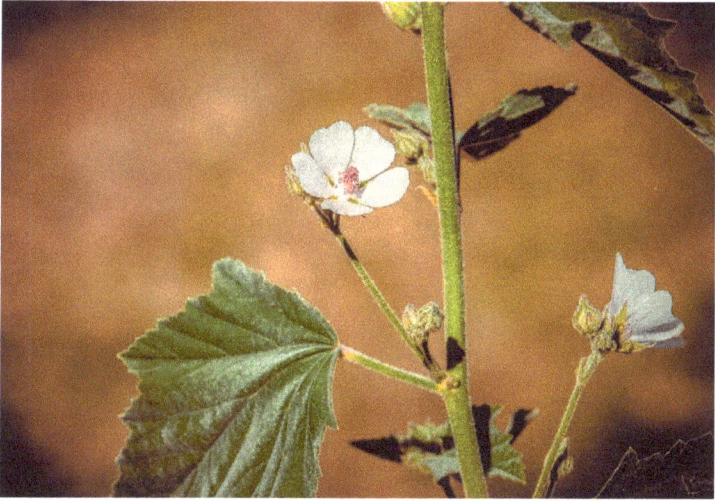

Meadowsweet *Filipendula ulmaria*

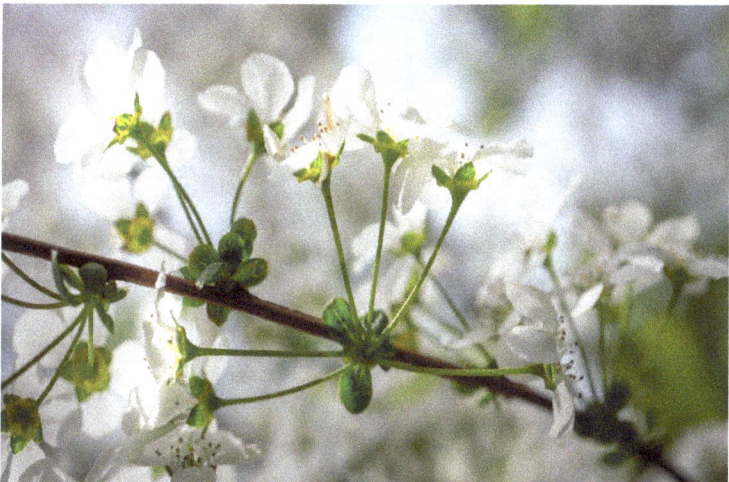

Meadowsweet

Filipendula ulmaria

For some women joint pain and menopause go hand in hand, meadowsweet may be of assistance if you are experiencing this.

If heartburn is interfering with your daily life, then give meadowsweet a try.

Meadowsweet may also be of assistance if you are having urine and bladder infections.

How to brew

Infusion: 2 tablespoons of fresh leaves and/or flowers per cup of boiling water or 1 tablespoon of dried leaves and/or flowers per cup of boiling water. Steep covered for 5-15 minutes

Decoction:

1. 2 tablespoons of crushed roots per cup of cold water, bring to boil, slow simmer for 5 minutes with lid on saucepan. Consume.

2. Soak crushed root in cold water for six hours, boil, strain, then consume.

Meadowsweet contains salicylic acid do not use if you react to salicylates. Do not use if you have an allergy to aspirin. People with asthma should not use without the consent of their health care professional as it may stimulate bronchial spasms.

Mint

Peppermint Mentha piperita

Spearmint Mentha spicata

Peppermint has a stronger flavour than spearmint and is usually the preferred mint for mint tea. Traditionally women have used mint to address hot flushes. Mint is also added to tea blends to improve the flavour.

The science about mint is somewhat lacking but we do know that spearmint has been identified as having the potential to assist women with PCOS.

Consumption of mint may assist with digestive issues.

How to brew

Infusion: 1 teaspoon of dried leaves or 3 teaspoons of fresh crushed leaves per cup of boiling water. Steep to taste. Mint is great in tea blends and may be consumed hot or cold.

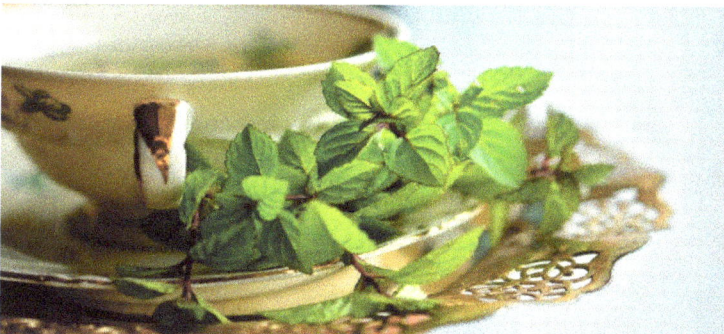

Consumption of mint may inhibit the uptake of iron so if you are being treated for iron deficiency or have low iron seek assistance from your health care professional before using mint to address menopausal symptoms.

Mistletoe

Viscum album

Viscum album is the European mistletoe. It is indicated for hot flushes, headaches, high blood pressure. It also may benefit sleep issues and relieve anxiety.

According to an animal study done in 2014, *Viscum album* may help with dyslipidaemia and muscle loss associated with menopause and post menopause.

Australian mistletoe, *Amyema spp.* have had little scientific study done to determine their use. The indigenous people used mistletoe to treat fever and genital inflammation.

How to brew

Infusion: 1 teaspoon of dried leaves or 2 teaspoon of crushed fresh leaves per cup of boiling water. Steep for 5-15 minutes.

Do not use the berries they are toxic.

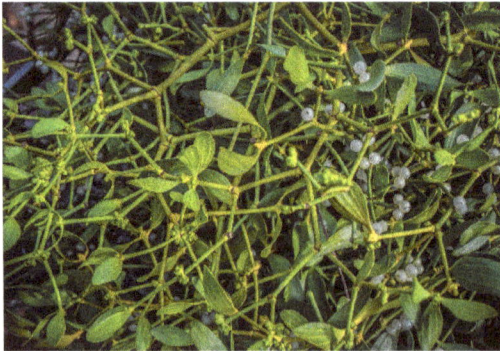

Do not use if pregnant or breastfeeding. Do not consume with alcohol or drugs for cold and flu with sedative, tranquilizers, barbiturates, muscle relaxants or medication for seizures. Do not use if you are taking blood pressure medication. If in doubt of what your medication does, please check with your health care professional before using mistletoe.

Moringa

Moringa oleifera

When experiencing hair loss during menopause use moringa both as a tea and as a hair rinse, you may find the iron and zinc constituents in moringa reduce fallout.

Moringa may also be of benefit if you are suffering from anaemia. Moringa may assist with headaches, constipation, and has the potential to increase your libido. Moringa tea has traditionally been used to assist with digestive issues.

How to brew

Use the freshest leaves, that is, the green leaves not the yellow ones. The leaves are then dried and crushed or ground into a powder. Store in a dark airtight container.

Infusion: ½ - ⅔ a teaspoon of moringa powder to 1 cup of boiling water. Stir and consume.

Some people prefer to drink moringa tea made with nut milk. Replace water with nut milk for a creamier texture.

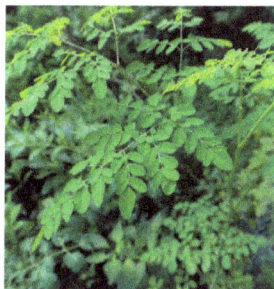

Moringa may lower blood sugar levels so diabetes may need to adjust insulin levels or consult with their health care professional before using. Moringa may have a laxative effect and may upset stomach if consumed in large amounts. One cup a day is enough. Do not use if pregnant.

Motherwort

Leonurus cardiaca

For the menopausal woman who is feeling anxious or depressed motherwort is worth considering. It can lower blood pressure, so if you have high blood pressure it may be a good choice for you.

Motherwort can assist with rapid heart rates.

Insomnia may improve when using motherwort. It is also used to address muscle spasm and menstrual cramping.

How to brew

Infusion: 1 tablespoon of dry leaves or 1 tablespoons of fresh crushed herbs per cup of boiling water, steep 5-10 minutes. This tea is bitter so a good option may be too included it in a blend with sweeter herbs.

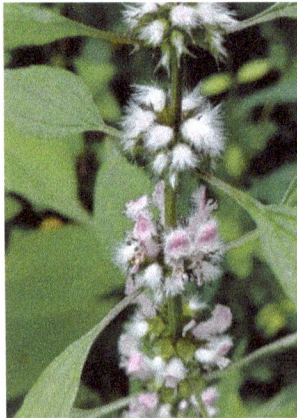

Do not use in pregnancy. Do not use if taking blood thinning medication. Do not use if you are experiencing heavy menstrual bleeding. Major interactions may occur with medications that are sedative, called CNS depressants, if you are taking these kinds of medications do not use motherwort. If you are unsure if your medication fits this category check with your health care professional before using motherwort.

Mugwort

Artemisia vulgari, Artemisia argyi, Artemisia douglasiana,

Artemisia california (sagebrush)

The first three mugworts above are used to assist women with hot flushes, anxiety, stress and depression. Mugwort may assist in boosting digestion and energy levels.

Artemisia california, sagebrush, along with other mugworts are consumed to help bring about dreaming in sleep. Dreaming is a natural part of the sleep cycle and is considered healthy. **Native North Americans used a decoction of *Artemisia california* to address menopause trauma.**

Artemisia vulgaris and *Artemisia argyi* are used to reduce bleeding in menopausal women.

How to brew

Infusion: 1 teaspoon of dried leaves and/or flowers or 3 teaspoon of fresh leaves and/or flowers per cup of boiling water. Steep 5-10 minutes.

Decoction: Root, leaves and flowers may be used. 30gms dried mugwort to one litre of water (4 cups). Boil water, then add mugwort, reduce heat to a slow simmer for 3 minutes, remove from heat, steep for 5 minutes then strain and consume.

Do not use if pregnant may induce an abortion. Not enough information is known about mugwort and breast feeding thus do not use. People allergic to birch, celery or wild carrot, royal jelly, honey, latex, peach kiwi fruit other Artemisia and sage should not use mugwort. If you are allergic to the Asteraceae/Compositae family do not use. Do not be tempted to use artemisia oil to make tea or add to your tea as ingestion of these oils may cause seizures and kidney damage.

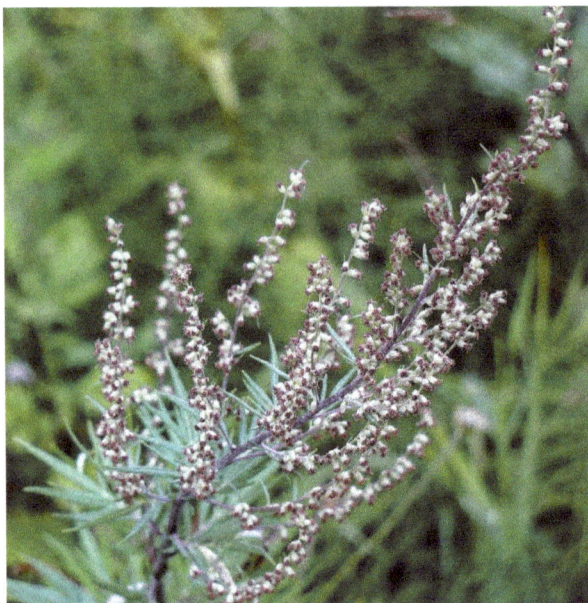

Mugwort

Nettle

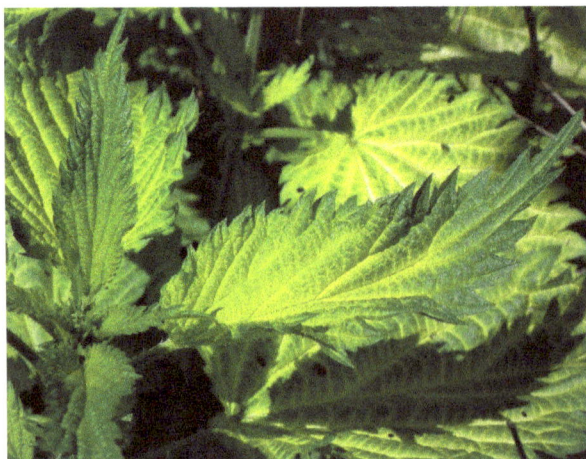

Mullein

Verbascum thapsus

More known for its ability to assist with respiratory disorders mullein may be of assistance to menopausal women suffering from incontinence as it may help to strengthen connective tissue in the urinary system. Some traditional sources used mullein leaves for address urinary tract infection. Today modern herbal medicine is more inclined to use the root.

Mullein may also assist with muscular pain and muscle tension. Some people drink the tea to assist with nervous tension and stress.

How to brew

Infusion: 1 teaspoon of dried or 3 teaspoons of crushed leaves and flowers or a teaspoon of chopped root per cup of boiling water. Steep 5-10 minutes. Strain well to remove fine hairs that cover the leaves.

Decoction: Use 1-2 teaspoons of chopped root per cup of water in your decoction. Simmer as per other herbs being used. Steep for 5 minutes. Strain and consume.

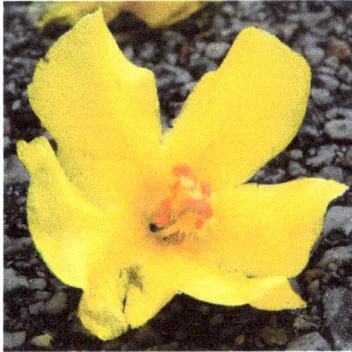

Apart from allergies not a lot is known about mullein interactions. It is advised not to take when pregnant.

Nettle

Urtica dioica

Nettle leaf tea is a powerhouse for menopausal women as it has the potential to regulate hormones, assist with hot flushes and night sweats, bloating, anxiety, poor sleep and insomnia.

Nettle has the capacity to assist with muscle tension, joint pain and menstrual cramping.

It is also used to address the most horrid menopausal symptoms, vaginal dryness, irritation and discharge. For these vaginal symptoms be sure to use the root of the nettle in a decoction.

This herb is a good consideration if you are experiencing any of these symptoms along with feeling fatigued.

Nettle is a good source of iron so if you are suffering from hair loss, anaemia or experiencing heavy bleeding it is worth considering.

How to brew

Infusion:

Option 1. Use 2 teaspoons of crushed dried leaves or 1-2 teaspoon of dried root per cup of boiling water. Steep 5-10 minutes.

Option 2. Warm a jar, (mason jars work well) with hot water. Add one cup of fresh leaves. Cover with cheesecloth. Let sit for 10 hours or overnight. Strain and consume over the next 48 hours. Store in refrigerator.

Some people may react to nettle tea just start with one cup to see how your body reacts on the first day.

Oak/White oak

Quercus alba

The bark of the white oak is used to make oak tea, it is often ground to a similar texture as coffee. Oak tea is not recommended for daily consumption but rather to address a particular issue, such as diarrhoea, pin worms or the loss of appetite.

Oak tea contains 15-20% tannins.

For the menopausal women oak tea may also assist with joint pain and urinary tract infections. Traditional used in conditions of weakened veins such as varicose veins and haemorrhoids.

How to brew

Infusion: Use 1 teaspoon of ground white oak inner bark per cup of boiling water. Steep for 5- 10 minutes.

Decoction: Boil 500ml of water in a saucepan add approximately 1 tablespoon of inner bark from the white oak tree and simmer for ten minutes. Remove and strain. Consume 1- 3 cups a day.

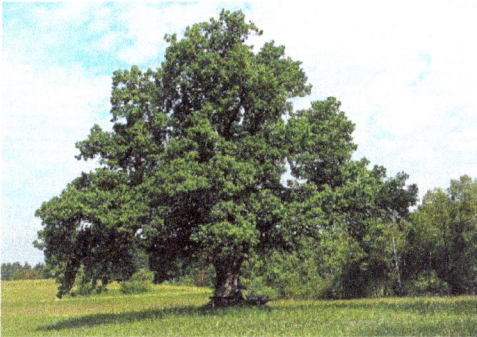

Do not use if pregnant or breastfeeding. Do not use if you have kidney or liver disorders or are taking medication to treat heart, kidney or liver conditions. Please check with your health care professional if taking other medications to ensure white oak is safe for you to consume.

Oats/Oats straw

Avena sativa

Oat tea is made from green oats. It has been used medicinally since the middle ages, if not before. Science has shown that oat straw has the potential to improve cognitive function.

For the menopausal woman oats may assist with anxiety, depression, stress, cramping or just feeling worn out.

How to brew

Infusion: In a jar place half a cup of green oat/oat straw per 500 ml of boing water. Put the lid on the jar or cover with a plate and steep for 8-10 hours. Strain and consume within 48 hours. Store in the refrigerator. Consider adding oat tea to other hot teas. Particularly good combined with lemon teas or ginger.

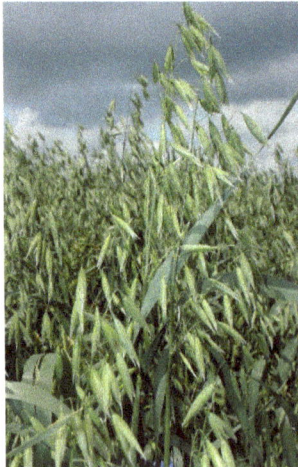

Oat tea is safe to use during pregnancy and is safe for children.

Orange Peel

Citrus X sinensis

Orange peel contains flavonoids and antioxidants and may assist the menopausal woman who is experiencing inflammation. As it contains hesperidin it may assist with the lowering of blood pressure and cholesterol levels.

Orange peel may also be of assistance to those suffering from headaches, nausea and constipation. It also contains some iron and vitamin C so if you are suffering from anaemia adding some orange peel to your tea may be of benefit.

The flavour of orange may enhance your tea blend and the peel may be consumed. Orange peel also contains volatile oils so inhale the vapour from your cup.

How to brew

Start with organic orange peel. Wash well. Dry it by leaving on the bench or in an oven.

Infusion: Use 1-2 teaspoons of dried orange peel per cup of boiling water. Steep 10-15 minutes.

Decoction: Use 1-2 tablespoon per 500ml of water. Bring water to boil simmer 5 minutes. Steep 10 minutes covered. Delicious hot or cold.

Cinnamon is often used in orange tea. Consider adding orange peel to your decoction blend.

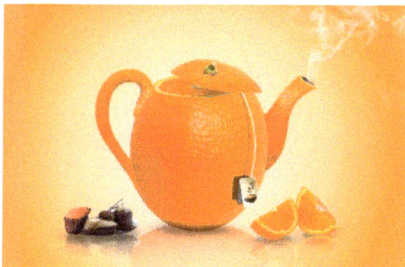

Oregano

Origanum vulgare

Oregano is sometimes called wild marjoram. This herb may be of assistance to the peri-menopausal women suffering from cramping. It is also used in digestive disorders including heart burn.

If suffering from candida (thrush), urinary tract infections then consider adding a cup or two of oregano to your daily regime.

Three cups a day should be plenty.

How to brew

Infusion: 1 teaspoon of dried herbs or 3 teaspoons of fresh crushed herbs per cup of boiling water. Steep for 5-10 minutes. Strain and consume.

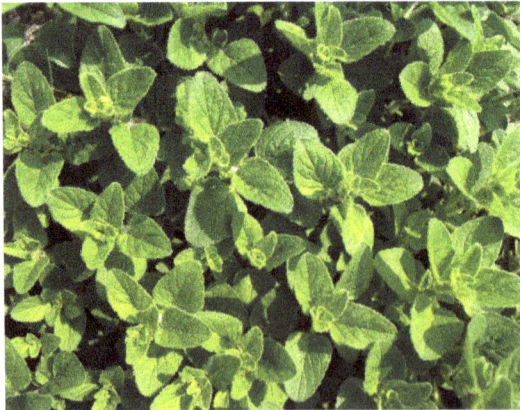

Considered generally safe in pregnancy. In high doses oregano may bring on uterine contractions, please seek advice from your health care professional if pregnant.

Parsley

Petroselinum crispum

Known as the blood toner parsley is a great tea to assist the peri-menopausal women with blood flow. If you are experiencing clotting, cramping and uneven flow when menstruating then give this tea a try.

Some women find parsley assists with bloating and constipation.

Parsley is traditionally used to address anxiety, headaches and UTI's.

How to brew

Infusion: 1 teaspoon of dried parsley or 3 teaspoons of fresh parsley per cup of off the boil water, this means let the kettle sit for a few minutes before you pour the water on the herbs. Steep for 5-20 minutes. Strain and consume.

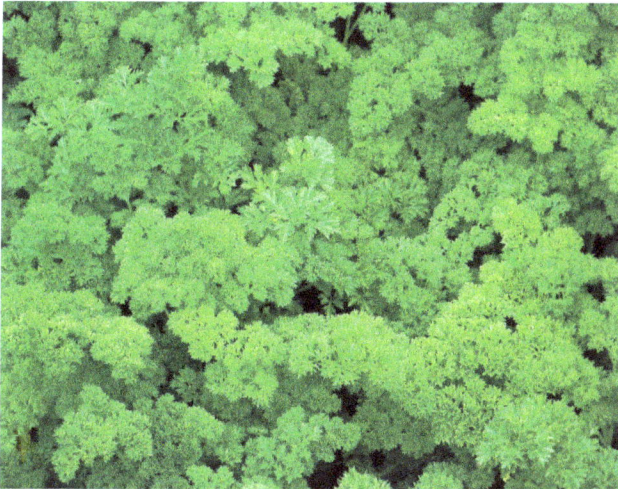

Parsley tea should not be consumed by pregnant women as it may stimulate the uterus. Do not use if you have kidney issues or taking medication treating kidney disorders. If unsure consult with your health care professional.

Passionflower

Passiflora incarnata

Passiflora edulis f. flavicarpa

Passionflower may assist the menopausal woman with hot flushes and nights sweats. Passionflower is often used by natural therapists to assist with anxiety and sleep issues.

Studies have shown that *Passiflora edulis f. flavicarpa* has the potential to reduce blood pressure. You may like to try using the peel of the actual fruit in your tea to assist with blood pressure.

How to brew

Infusion: 1 teaspoon of dried leaves or 3 teaspoons of chopped fresh leaves and flowers per cup of boiling water.

Peel may be added either grated or cut into pieces. Remember to wash peel before using. Steep for 10 minutes. Strain and consume.

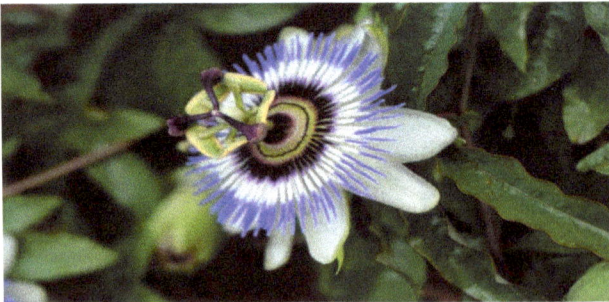

Check with your health care professional before using passionflower if you are on blood pressure medication and do not come off blood pressure medication to substitute with passionflower without talking to your health care professional.

Pau D'arco

Handroanthus impetiginosus

Tabebuia impetiginosa

Commonly referred to as the pink trumpet tree. The inner bark of the tree has been identified as having antibacterial and anti-inflammatory actions. Traditional uses of Pau D'arco include treating cystitis, cervical inflammation and to assist with lowering blood pressure.

Pau D'arco also contains the mineral calcium and silica which may assist with bone health.

How to brew

Decoction: Crush the bark in a pestle and mortar (or food processor). Place in a glass or ceramic bowl and cover with boiling water about 3 cm above the herb, soak overnight. In the morning place into a saucepan add water to cover 3 cm above herb. Bring to boil, reduce heat to a gentle simmer for 20 minutes. Strain through a sieve or cheese cloth. Discard the bark and consume the tea within 2-3 days. Store in the refrigerator.

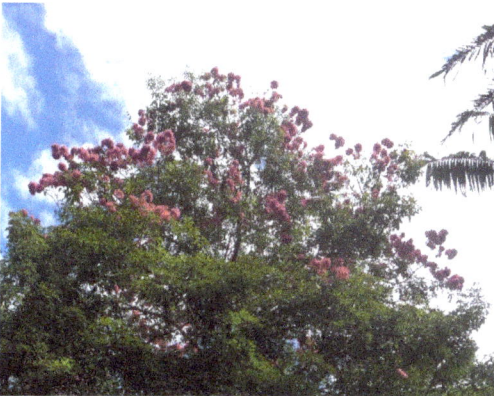

Peony

Paeonia officinalis (Red)

Paeonia lactiflora (white)

Peony root tea is another tea that may benefit women with PCOS, but it is also great for other symptoms of menopausal women. It may be of assistance to women who are feeling moody, fatigued and those who are experiencing migraines

Some women take peony to address heavy bleeding and painful menstruation due to its ability to assist with cramping as well as providing relief from headaches, dizziness and tinnitus.

Peony may also have the potential to improve arthritis symptoms. Tea made from the flowers and leaves of the peony is used traditionally to treat haemorrhoids and varicose veins.

How to brew

Infusion: Use 3-4 teaspoons of fresh leaves or 2 teaspoons of dried root powder per cup of boiling water, steep 3-5 minutes.

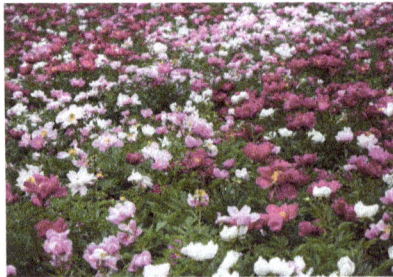

Peony reduces blood clotting ability so do not use if taking blood thinning medication or if you have blood disorders without consulting your health care professional. Cease using two weeks before surgery. Do not use if pregnant.

Plantain/Ribwort

Plantago major

Plantago lanceolata

Not to be confused with *Musa paradisaca* which is a type of banana also known as plantain.

Plantain is an herb to consider if you are experiencing heavy bleeding and menstrual cramping.

Plantain may be added to your bladder or urinary tract infection blend or taken alone.

How to brew

Infusion: Use 1 tablespoon of dried plantain or 3 tablespoons of fresh leaves per cup of boiling water. Steep covered for 20 minutes. May be refrigerated and kept for up to 48hrs.

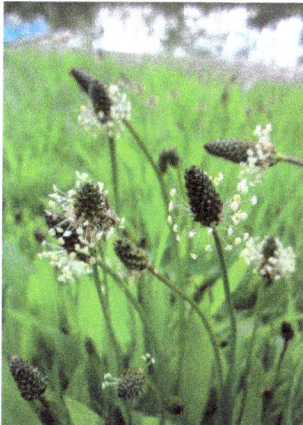

Do not use if pregnant May interact with lithium or carbamazepine.

Raspberry leaf

Rubus idaeus

Traditionally used for uterine health, containing both calcium and magnesium raspberry leaf tea may assist the peri-menopausal woman who is experiencing heavy bleeding and irregular periods. Raspberry leaf tea may assist in reducing severity of bleeds and pain associated with menstruation. Raspberry leaf may assist with modulating oestrogen and toning the uterus.

Fibroids may also be assisted using raspberry leaf tea.

How to brew

Infusion 1 teaspoon of dried leave or 3 teaspoons of fresh leaves per cup of boiling water. Steep to taste.

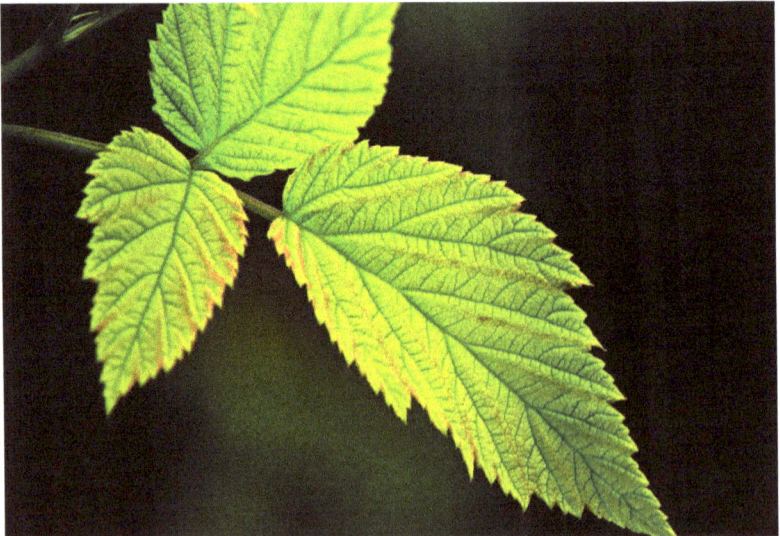

Not recommended for first trimester of pregnancy. Used later in pregnancy to prepare uterus for delivery.

Red Clover

Trifolium pratense

Red clover has been used by American Indians, in Chinese medicine and Ayurvedic medicine to address menopausal symptoms.

Red clover is used to address hot flushes and breast tenderness.

The science is inconclusive on its effects, this is partly due to the poor quality of the studies undertaken.

Clinical trials have identified that it has the potential to reduce hot flushes when used for 3-4 months. Red clover has been identified as containing phytoestrogenic isoflavones, which could contribute to these results.

How to brew

Red clover tea is made from the flowers and upper leaves. Harvest in early morning and avoid bruising the flower, when dried flowers will retain their colour.

Infusion: Use 2 flower heads or 2 teaspoons of head and leaves to one cup of boiled water. Steep for 10 minutes.

Cold tea: Use one cup of dried red clover, cover with one litre of water, boiled then cooled for 3 minutes. Steep for 8 hrs, strain and refrigerate. Consume within 48 hrs.

Do not use if pregnant or breastfeeding. If you have a hormone sensitive condition, have protein S deficiency and stop taking 2 weeks prior to surgery as it may reduce blood clotting ability.

If you are using medication to slow blood clotting or medication that are broken down in the liver. If you are on the oral contraceptive pill, please consult your health care professional before using red clover.

Tea for Menopause

Red clover, *Trifolium pratense*

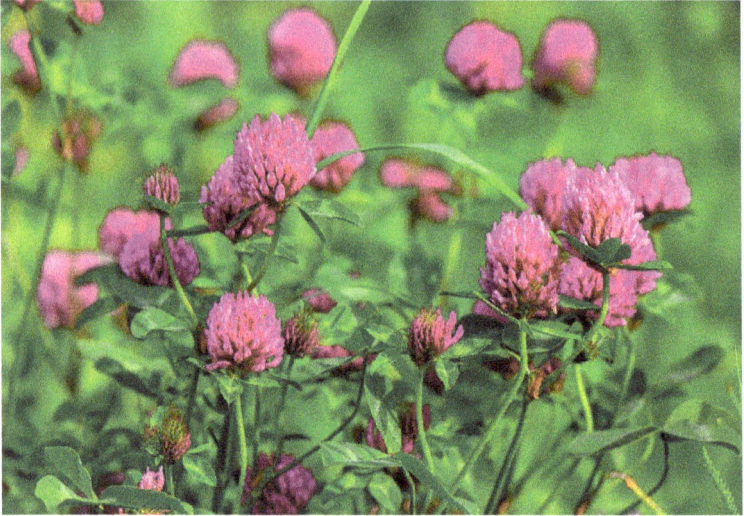

Rose, *Rosa ssp.*

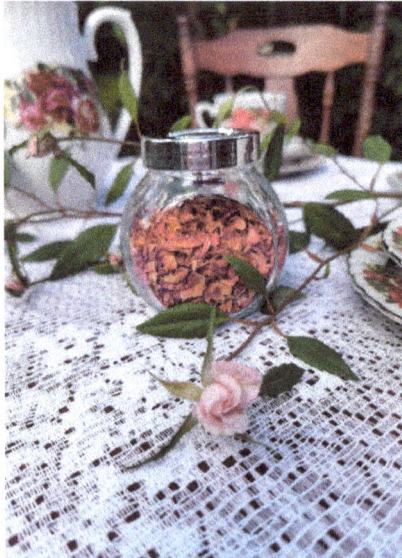

Rose

Rosa ssp.

Rose tea may help lift your mood, depression and reduce insomnia, it also may be of benefit if you are suffering from menstrual cramping or arthritis.

Rose tea assists may stimulate bile production which may assist with digestion. It has a mild laxative capacity.

Rose tea may assist in weight loss by assisting the body remove toxins. It is also a good consideration for urinary tract infections.

Rosebud tea contains caffeine ranging from a third to approximately half the amount a cup of coffee has, so if you are trying to reduce your caffeine intake rosebud tea may be a good substitute.

How to brew

Rose tea may be drunk alone, or you may choose to add a few buds to your other teas. The flowers are edible and have a velvety texture. Wash well before use.

Infusion: 1 teaspoon of dried rose petals or 3 teaspoons of fresh rose petals per cup of boiling water. Steep for a few minutes and consume.

Decoction: Add rose flowers or petals at the simmering or steeping stage, do not boil them.

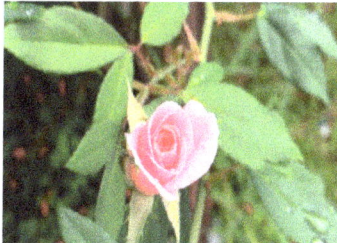

Roselle

Hibiscus sabdariffa

The flower of the Roselle is called the calyx and is used to make tea. Traditionally used to treat high blood pressure and heart disease. Human studies have shown that roselle tea has the potential to reduce blood pressure in adults with mild hypertension

Roselle has some phytoestrogenic properties which may assist the peri-menopausal experience irregular periods and menstrual cramping.

Roselle has been used to treat anxiety and depression in traditional Mexican medicine.

While for some people roselle alleviates digestive issues, for others a side effect of roselle may be upset stomach. If this occurs cut back or cease using.

How to brew

Infusion: 1 tablespoon of fresh petals to 1 cup of boiling water, steep 3-5 minutes, strain and consume.

Cold infusion: 1-2 tablespoons of fresh petals per cup of cold water, filtered or spring is best, cover and steep for 4-6 hours. Strain and consume. Refrigerate if desired.

Decoction: Place 5 cups of fresh flower petals or 1/2 a cup of dried crushed flowers in 2 litres of cold water in a saucepan bring to boil, turn off heat, add other flavours such as lemon or lime zest steep of approximately 20 minutes. Strain and consume. May be served hot or cold. Store in the refrigerator.

The effect of Roselle tea is unknown for pregnant and breastfeeding. Do not use if suffering or being treated for low blood pressure or if you are taking blood pressure medication without consulting your health care professional. Interacts with acetaminophen, do not use if taking this medication without medical advice. Diabetes note roselle may decrease blood sugar levels. Consult with your health care professional.

Tea for Menopause

Roselle

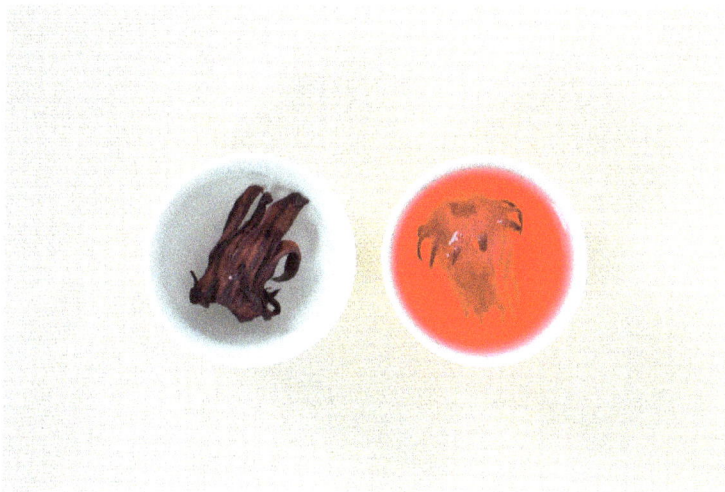

Rosemary.

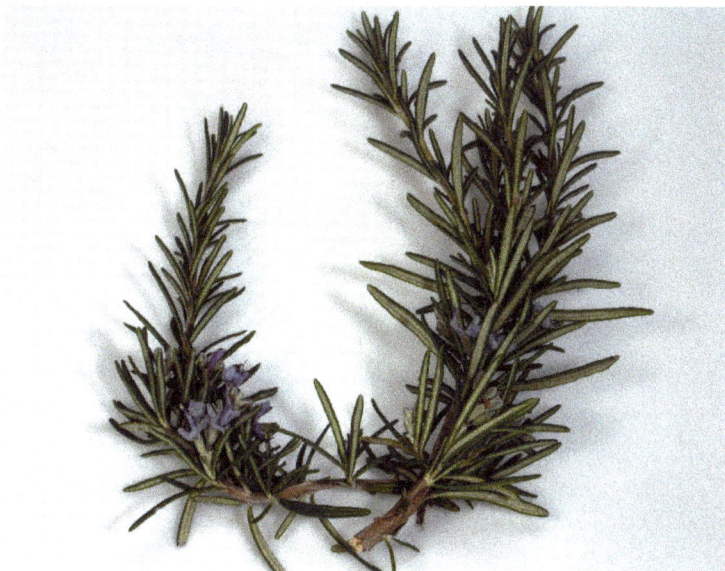

Rosemary

Salvia rosmarinus, Rosmarinus officinalis

Do you have rosemary growing in your garden? Have you ever made a tea with it? If not, maybe it's time to give it a try! Rosemary may assist those suffering with anxiety and depression. It helps with memory including forgetfulness and lifting that dreaded brain fog.

It may also relieve muscle tension and assist with sleep.

How to brew

Infusion:

Flowers: 1 teaspoon of dried herb or 3 teaspoons of fresh herb per cup of boiling water. Steep 5 minutes.

Leaves (stronger flavour): 1/2 teaspoon of dried leaves or fresh leaves per cup of boiling water. Steep to taste.

Particularly delicious with a piece of lemon.

Decoction:

When boiling a decoction for ten or more minutes the whole stem may be used. For shorter decoctions that are just brought to boil then simmered use the green sprigs or leaves. Remove stem before consuming.

Do not use if pregnant and breastfeeding. Do not use if taking blood thinning medication, using diuretic medication or if you are taking lithium. If unsure if rosemary will interact with your medication, please consult your health care provider. If you are allergic to aspirin or react to salicylates avoid rosemary. If you suffer from seizures rosemary should not be used.

Saffron

Crocus sativus

Saffron may assist with mood, anxiety and depression in some people.

It is great to assist memory and is used for menstrual cramping. Large doses of saffron are poisonous. Quantities over 5 grams per day are potential harmful, over 12 grams may be fatal.

How to brew

Infusion: Place 3 or 4 strands of saffron in cup or tea pot add 2-3 cm of warm water, steep for 10 minutes then add boiling water. Saffron can be added to other tea, just add 1 or 2 strands per cup.

Decoction: Saffron may be used along with other herbs including cinnamon, ginger, mint and lemon.

Saffron may assist with anxiety and depression but it may also make them worse in some people especially those with dipolar disorder so if you have bipolar or feel worse after using saffron do not use and seek medical attention if required.

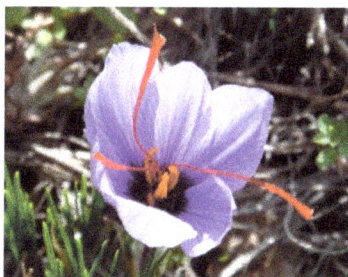

Do not use in pregnancy and breast feeding. Do not use if allergic to Lolium, Olea and Salsola plant species. If you have a heart condition or suffer from low blood pressure do not use without consultation with a health care professional.

Sage

Salvia officinalis

Hot flushes and night sweats, mental fatigue and weight gain are symptoms that sage may benefit.

Sage tea may assist if your bladder is overactive, meaning you constantly need to urinate.

It may also assist if you are feeling down and anxious.

Sage tea may assist with appetite for those of you who are feeling off their food.

How to brew

Infusion: Use one teaspoon of dried or 2 teaspoons of freshly chopped leaves and tops per cup of boiling water. Cover and steep for 5-10 minutes. Strain and consume.

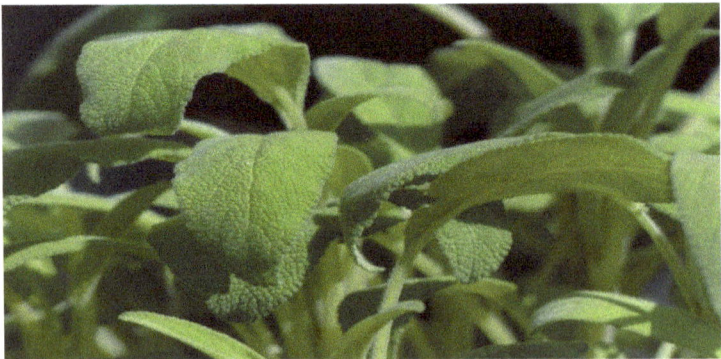

Do not drink more than 5 cups of sage tea a day, as sage contains thujones and camphor which are not recommended in large quantities. Do not use if you suffer from seizures. Do not use if you have an estrogen reactive cancer, if in doubt consult your health care professional. Do not use if you have a liver or kidney disorder unless cleared by a health care professional.

Sarsaparilla

Smilax spp /Smilax Ornate

Do not confuse sarsaparilla with Indian sarsaparilla *Hemidesmus indicus* as it doesn't have the same active ingredients as the smilax *spp.* does.

Sarsaparilla may be of assistance to menopausal women with muscle tension, headaches or are feeling fatigued.

Sarsaparilla may assist with detoxification of the liver and hormone function.

Sarsaparilla has traditionally been used to increase libido.

How to brew

Infusion: Add 2 teaspoon of ground fresh root or 1 teaspoon of dried crush root or root powder to one cup of boiling water, stir and steep for 5-10 minutes.

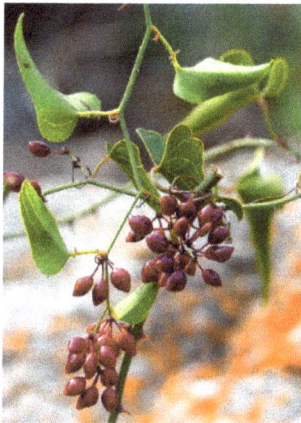

Safety in pregnancy and breastfeeding has not been established, best not to use without medical advice. If on medication, please check with your health care professional before using sarsaparilla.

Saw Palmetto

Serenoa repens

Saw palmetto is used to address PCOS and other hormone imbalances which involve oestrogen and testosterone. It is used to address genitourinary health in both sexes as well as libido. If you are experiencing a low sex drive, urinary tract infection or urinary incontinence then give saw palmetto a try.

It is also being used to address hair loss and baldness.

How to brew

Decoction: Use 1 teaspoon of crushed berries per cup of water. Place water and berries in a saucepan on low heat and slowly bring to boil and simmer for 10 minutes with lid on.

Strain and consume.

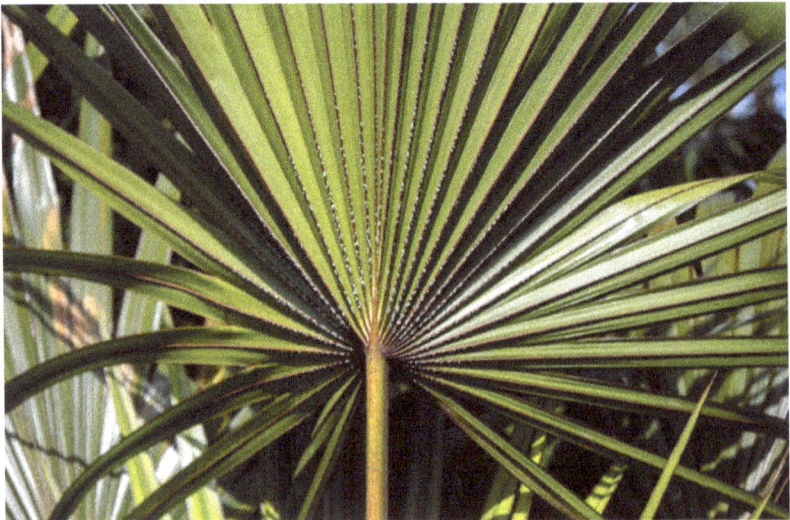

Sea buckthorn

Hippophae rhomboids

Both seeds and leaves can be used to make sea buckthorn tea. The oil in the berries has been studied and shown to assist with menopause and postmenopausal virginal dryness, itching and burning.

Sea buckthorn tea may assist with weight loss. Studies in mice have shown that tea made from the leaves reduced visceral fat.

How to brew

Berry Infusion: Place 50 gram of whole berries per cup into a heat proof container. Crush the berries releasing the juice. Pour boiling water on top of berries and juice and steep 5-10 minutes. Some people like to add a cinnamon stick to the tea. Just add before pouring in water. 3-5 cm stick is fine.

Leaf Infusion: Use the leaves from the male plant. Only female plants bear the berries. The leaves are usually dried before being made into tea. Use 1 teaspoon of dried leaves per cup of boiling water. Steep for 5-10 minutes.

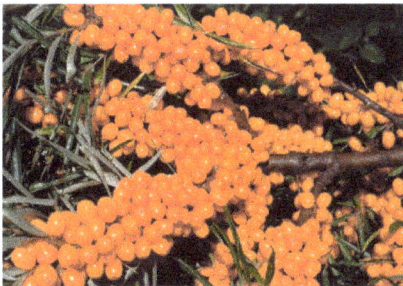

Do not use if on medications that thins your blood or slows blood clotting. These include aspirin and warfarin. If unsure check with your health care professional. It is believed that sea buckthorn may lower blood pressure. No information on safety in pregnancy of breastfeeding available, Stop using 2 weeks before surgery.

Senna

Senna alexandrina, Cassia acutifolia

Senna tea is used to treat constipation and for weight loss due to its ability to cleanse the colon. As a side effect you may experience cramping and abdominal pain.

Using senna for weight loss is not recommended as it moves food too quickly through the intestine, which means the nutrients required are moved through before they can be absorbed completely by the body.

Senna is a laxative and great for occasional use. If you are suffering from regular bouts of constipation, please see your health care professional to develop a treatment plan.

How to brew

Infusion: Use 1/4 of a teaspoon of crushed leaves per cup of just off the boil water. Steep for 10 minutes. Strain and consume.

Try drinking Senna tea in the evening so bowel movements occur in the morning. Do not use large amounts of senna as diarrhoea and stomach cramps may result.

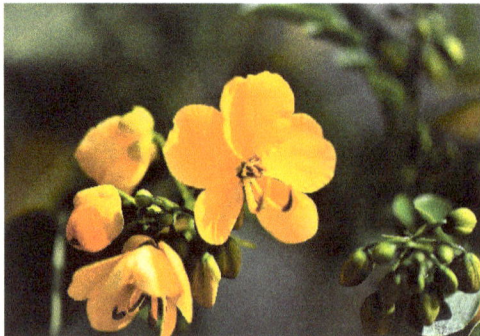

It is recommended that you do not use senna for more than two weeks.

Sheep's Sorrel

Rumex acetosella

Also known as Red Sorrel. Do not confuse *Rumex acetosella* and Roselle (*Hibiscus sabdariffa*). Both are sometimes referred to as Sorrel, check your botanical name when purchasing product.

Sorrel may help with hair loss during menopause. It is also indicated for digestive issues and weight loss especially if you have obesity issues.

Sorrel is one of four herbs in Essiac tea which was traditionally used in addressing cancer but today is more commonly used for detoxing.

How to brew

Infusion: Use ¼ of a cup of sorrel fresh leaves per cup of boiling water. Steep 5-10 minutes. Strain and consume.

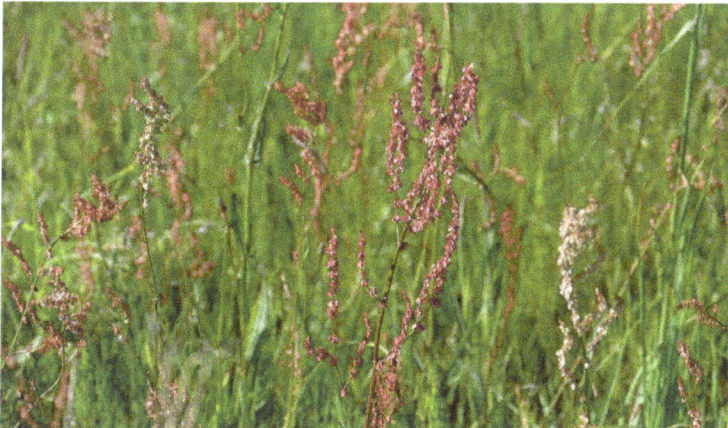

Do not use if pregnant. If on medication check with your health care professional before using sorrel. Sorrel may lower blood pressure. Stop use two weeks before surgery.

Shepherd's purse

Capsella bursa-pastoris

Traditionally Shepherd's purse was and still is used by women to address excessive menstrual bleeding and cramping.

Shepherd's purse has been identified as having anti-inflammatory and anti-oxidative benefits in animal studies.

It may also assist digestion and headaches.

Shepherd's purse is so named because the heart shaped seed pods resembled the purses shepherds carried their valuables in when tending their flocks.

How to brew

Infusion: Use 1-3 heaped teaspoons of dried leaves, stems and flowers per cup of boiling water. Steep for 15 minutes. Consume.

Shepherd purse is often combined with yarrow to address heavy bleeding.

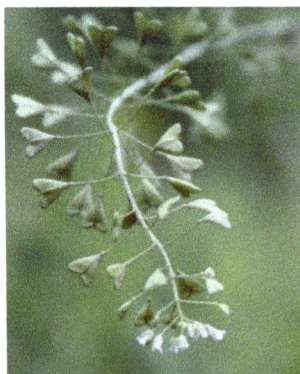

Do not use if pregnant or breastfeeding. Some people are allergic to shepherds' purse, if using for first time use a low dose. Check with your health care professional if on medication to see if it is a tea you should be using.

Skullcap

Scutellaria lateriflora

Feeling depressed and moody or anxious then skullcap is a tea to consider. It appears that skullcap may have the potential to calm the over thinking minds of women with menopause.

Skullcap is also used to address sleep issues and headaches.

Skullcap is traditionally used to address muscle spasm and restless legs.

How to brew

Infusion: 1 teaspoon of dried herb or 2 teaspoons of fresh herb per cup of boiling water. Add off the boil water to herbs and cover and steep for 5-10 minutes.

Consume one hour before bed to assist with sleep. Recommended daily dose of skullcap is between 6-15 gm for an adult. Do not exceed this dosage.

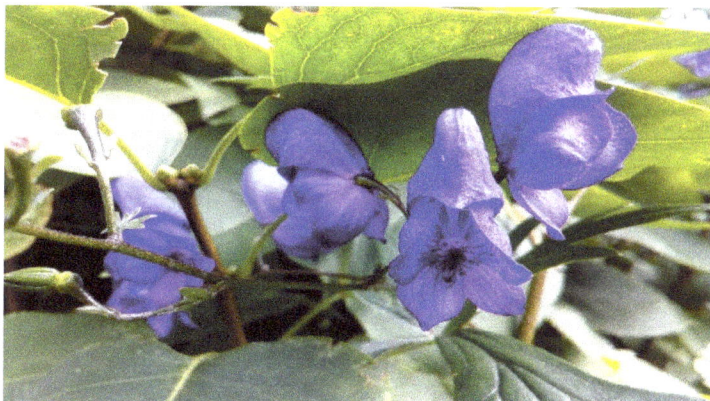

Not enough research to know how safe skullcap is in pregnancy or breastfeeding thus it is advised to avoid use. Stop using two weeks prior to surgery as there is some concern it may slow down the nervous system and interfere with anaesthesia.

Solomons seal

Polygonatum biflorum

Solomons seal was traditionally used and is still used today to assist with hot flushes and mood issues. For some women its biggest benefit is with addressing vaginal irritation and dryness. This is an herb you may wish to include in your down below blend.

Some natural therapists refer to Solomons seal as the joint juice due to its potential to assist with joint pain associated with arthritis.

How to brew

Hot Infusion: ½ a teaspoon of chopped root per cup of boiling water. Steep 10 minutes. Root will swell in the bottom of cup, so you don't need to strain unless you wish to.

Cold Infusion: Place ½ a teaspoon of chopped root into a cup or jar with one cup of cold water cover with a lid or cloth and sit at room temperature overnight. In the morning heat and consume or refrigerate until ready to consume. Keeps for 48 hours.

Do not consume more than 3 cups a day. You may find one is enough.

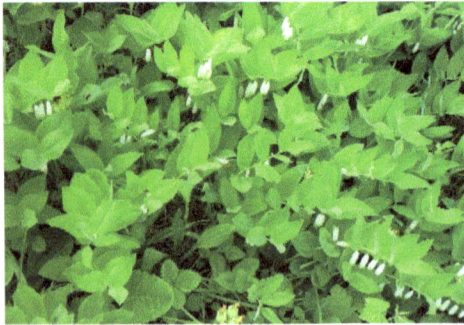

Do not use if you're are pregnant, on medication to lower your blood pressure or have low blood pressure or if you are on heart medication without first checking with your treating health care professional.

Southernwood

Artemisia abrotanum

Southernwood is one herb which has traditionally been used to treat urinary tract infections, menstrual cramping, insomnia and digestive issues.

Modern research has identified Southernwood tea has the potential to boost the immune system.

Southernwood has a fragrance similar to camphor and has been use for centuries to repel moths and other insects.

How to brew

Infusion: Use 1 teaspoon of dried herb per cup of boiling water. Steep 5-10 minutes.

Consumption of 1 or 2 cups a day is recommended.

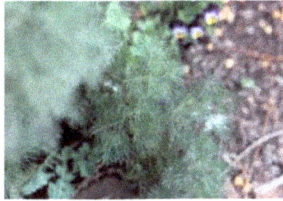

Do not use if pregnant as it may cause uterine contractions and miscarriages. If you are taking medications, please consult your health care professional before using southernwood.

St John's Wort

Hypericum perforatum

St John's wort is used to address depression and may assist with anxiety, mood swings and insomnia. It also has the potential to reduce the frequency and duration of hot flushes.

Relieving muscle and nerve pain in another reason people drink St John's wort.

St John's wort is often combined with black cohosh to address menopausal symptoms.

How to brew

Infusion: Use 2 teaspoons of fresh leaves and flowers or 1 teaspoon of dried leaves and flowers per cup of boiling water. Steep for 5-10 minutes. Strain and consume.

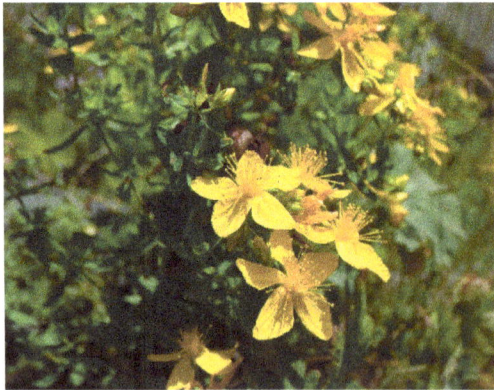

St John's wort is not recommended for people with severe depression. St John's wort is contraindicated for many medications so please check if you are on medication with your health care professional before using. St John's wort may induce photosensitivity in some people. Stop using two weeks prior to surgery as it may interfere with anaesthesia. Do not use if pregnant or breast feeding without consulting your health care professional.

St Mary's thistle

Silybum marianum

St Mary's thistle contains silymarin which is proven to be beneficial to the liver. It is accredited with having a detoxifying effect. Studies have identified St Mary's thistle as being of benefit in the reduction of hot flushes. This may be due its oestrogenic properties.

Traditionally used to assist with mood and depression.

May reduce the risk of oestrogen deficiency bone loss including osteoporosis.

How to brew

Infusion: 1 teaspoon of dried leaves or 3 heaped teaspoons of fresh leaves per cup of boiling water. Steep 10 minutes.

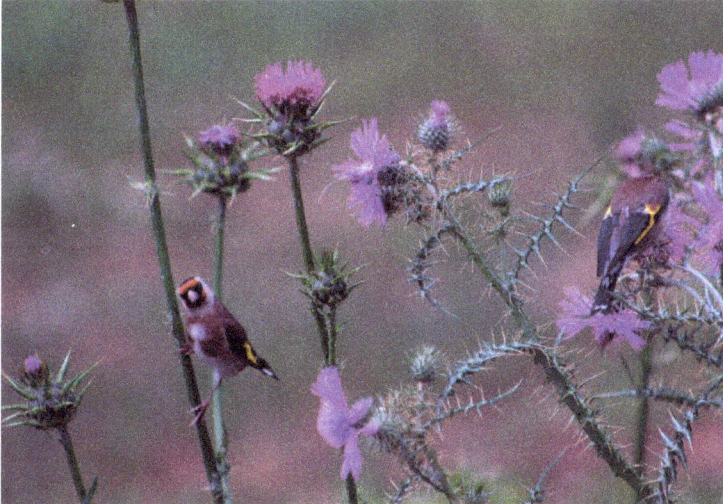

Diabetics should not use St Mary's thistle without the direction of a health care professional. Do not use if on blood thinning medication, taking statins or on medication for hypoglycaemia or depression without consulting your health care professional.

Summer Savory

Satureja hortensis

Summer savory may assist if you are feeling nauseous or are suffering from indigestion and gas. It may also assist with improving appetite.

It has traditionally been used to increase libido.

Summer savory is part of the mint family and its flavour is similar to thyme and oregano.

How to brew

Infusion: Use 1 teaspoon of dried leaves or 3 teaspoons of fresh crushed leaves per cup of boiling water. Steep 5-10 minutes.

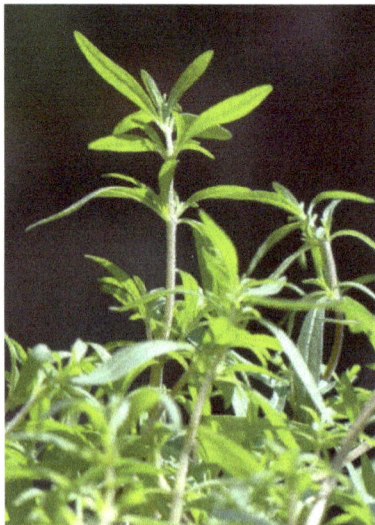

May slow blood clotting, do not use if you are taking medication for bleeding disorders. Stop use 2 weeks before surgery.

Tarragon

Artemisia dracunculus

Tarragon may assist women with digestive issue.

Not sleeping then the calming effect of tarragon may assist your sleep.

Tarragon is a natural antioxidant, which has a slightly bittersweet flavour and some people compare it to anise.

How to brew

Infusion: 1 tablespoon of fresh leaves or 1-2 teaspoons of dried leaves per cup of boiling water. Steep 5-10 minutes.

Ginger or mint are often used with tarragon.

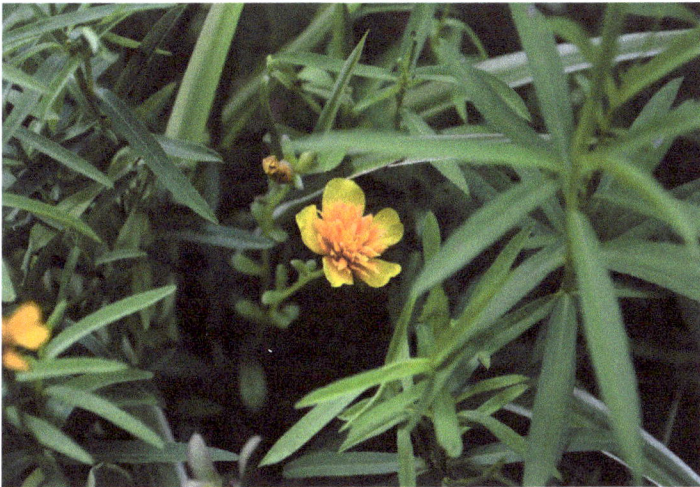

Do not consume in medicinal quantities if pregnant. Do not use if you have a bleeding disorder. If you are allergic to the Asteraceae/Compositae family which includes ragweed, chrysanthemums, marigolds, daisies etc. you have the possibility of also being allergic to tarragon, please check with your health care provider before using it.

117

Thyme

Thymus vulgaris

Thyme may be of assistance with bloating and digestive issues and may assist with lack of appetite.

Thyme is also used to assist with nervous tension, sleep issues and insomnia.

Thyme may also be beneficial for women experiencing menstrual and joint pain. It may also help regulate menstrual cycles.

How to brew

Infusion: Use leaves and tops. 1 teaspoon of dried herb or 3 teaspoons of fresh herbs per cup of boiling water. Steep for 10 minutes. Strain and consume.

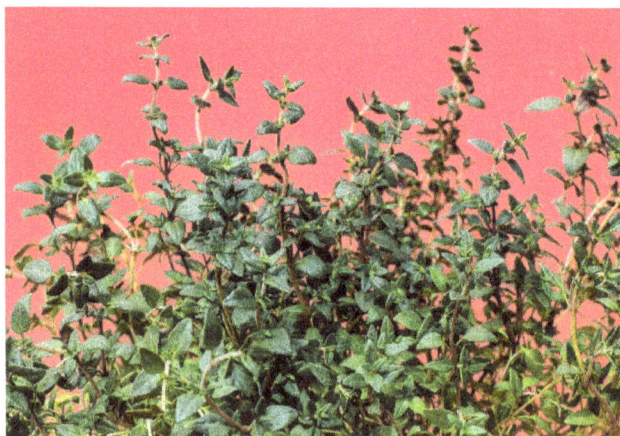

There is no research into the safety of thyme tea in pregnancy. People allergic to the Lamiaceae species may also be allergic to thyme. If you have a hormone sensitive condition or are taking hormone medication, please check with your health care professional before use. Do not use if you have a bleeding disorder, Thyme may slow blood clotting. Stop use 2 weeks prior to surgery.

Tribulus

Tribulus terrestris

If experiencing difficulties in the intimacy department, then tribulus may be the herb for you. Lack of desire, comfort and disinterest in foreplay may be improved with this tea.

Hot flushes and night sweats and fatigue also have the potential to be reduced by tribulus.

Tribulus is also used to address digestive issues and constipation. It may be of assistance if you are experiencing mood swings.

How to brew

Dry the young leaves of the tribulus plant, crush and store in a dark airtight container.

Infusion: Use 1 teaspoon of dried herb per cup of boiling water. Steep 5-10 minutes. Consume.

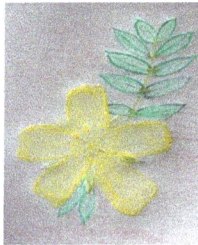

Do not use if pregnant or breast feeding. If you have prostate issues, have kidney disorders, or are diabetic do not use without first consulting with your health care professional. If you are on medication, please check with your health care professional as tribulus may interact with medications. Stop use 2 weeks prior to surgery.

Turmeric

Curcuma longa

For hot flushes, night sweats and mood swings. Try adding ¼ to ½ a teaspoon of organic turmeric powder to your tea blend.

Turmeric may be of assistance in addressing vaginal irritation and discharge. Turmeric may also assist in reduction of fat cells so may be of benefit for women experiencing menopausal weight gain.

How to brew

Infusion: ¼ - ½ teaspoon of powdered turmeric or ½ -1 teaspoon of grated fresh turmeric per cup of boiling water. Combines well with mint and lemon.

Decoction: In a saucepan place a 2 cm piece of fresh turmeric which has been cut thinly or grated with 2 cups of cold water and a dash of black pepper. Bring to boil and simmer for 5-8 minutes. Strain and consume.

Ginger may also be added to turmeric tea. The black pepper helps with the absorption of the constituent, curcumin in the turmeric.

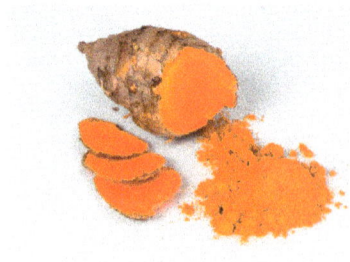

Do not use turmeric if you have gallbladder issues or gallstones. Turmeric may reduce blood clotting, do not use if you have bleeding disorders or on medication that thins your blood without the consent of your health care provider. Turmeric may reduce blood sugar levels in people with diabetes, check with your health care provider if concerned as to whether turmeric is right for you.

Valerian

Valeriana officinalis

Hot flushes and night sweats can make life hell, valerian to the rescue! Traditionally used to address these Symptoms, now with the science to back up! Definitely a tea to try.

Valerian is also used to assist with sleep and is traditionally used for anxiety and depression.

How to brew

Infusion: ½ teaspoon of dried root, either ground or powdered per cup of boiling water. Steep for 10 minutes. Strain and consume.

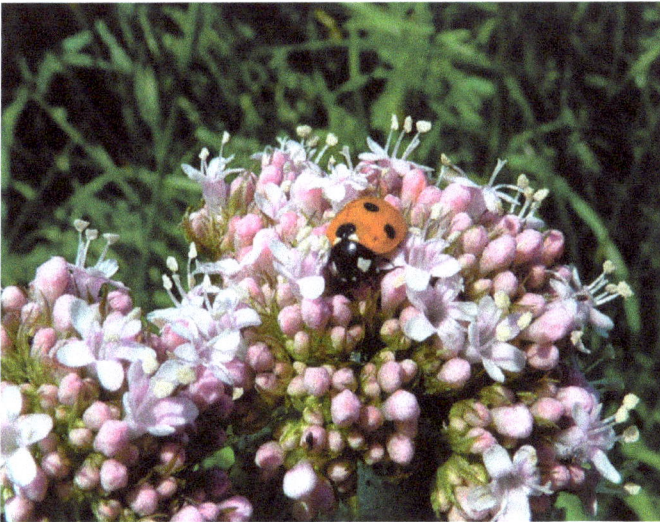

Do not consume alcohol and large amounts of valerian together as they doth induce sleepiness. Do not use valerian without consulting your health care professional if using medication that is sedative or induces drowsiness. If unsure of what your medications actions are check with a health care professional.

Verbena

Verbena officinalisa

Verbena is a tea to consider if you are suffering from headaches and migraines.

Joint aches, pains and menstrual cramps also may be assisted by consumption of verbena.

If you're feeling groggy and mentally fatigued, then you may wish to try verbena.

How to brew

Infusion: Use 4-6 fresh leaves or 1 teaspoon of dried leaf per cup of boiling water. Cover and steep for 5 minutes. Strain and consume.

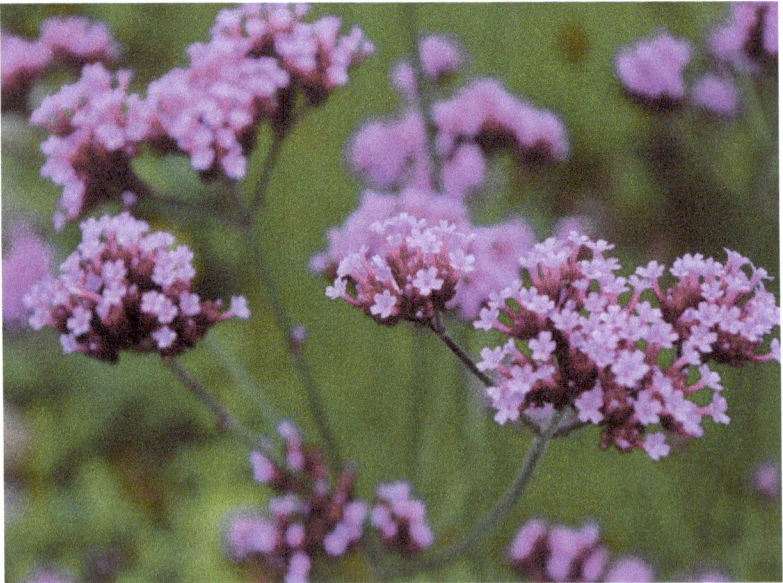

Vitex

Vitex agnus-castus

Also known as Chaste tree, vitex is used by menopausal women to assist with hot flushes, bloating and menstrual cramping. Vitex may also benefit women with fibroids which are another cause of increased vaginal bleeding during the menopausal years.

It may also be used to assist with sleep and mood swings.

Vitex may be able to reduce menopausal acne in some women.

Some women report bloating and weight gain from using vitex, if this occurs, try another tea.

How to brew

Infusion: 1 teaspoon of crushed berry per cup of boiling water. Steep for 10 minutes. May be enjoyed hot or cold.

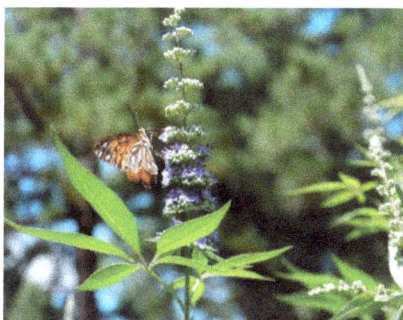

Do not use if pregnant or breastfeeding. Do not use if taking medication for Parkinson's disease. Do not use if taking antipsychotic drugs. Vitex will interact with some birth control pills, please check with your health care provider to check whether vitex is a good fit for you if using birth control. If on other medication check with your health care provider for possible interactions.

Wild Yam

Dioscorea villosa

Wild yam contains phytoestrogenic properties and many women have used wild yam to assist with menopausal symptoms including cramping and joint pain.

Diosgenin is a steroid compound that is used in the synthesis of steroid hormones including estrogen, progesterone and cortisol. It helps reduce inflammation and animal studies have shown it may benefit with the treatment of diabetes and arthritis. *Dioscorea villosa* has one of the highest levels of diosgenin of the 600 Dioscorea species.

Some women find that wild yam assists with urinary tract conditions this may be due to its diuretic and antispasmodic actions.

How to brew

Decoction: 1/2- 1 teaspoon of dried root powder per cup of water, simmer for 10 minutes. Consume only drink one cup a day.

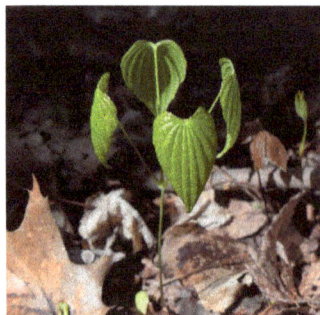

Wild yam may interfere with birth control pills, seek advice from your health care professional before use if on birth control. Do not use if pregnant or give to children without consulting a health care practitioner. Do not use if you have endometriosis, fibroids or cancer without first consulting your health care professional.

Willow

Salix alba

Black tea and willow bark tea both have a tannin content of around 13% giving them both a bitter taste, which makes them both good antioxidant teas. This may be one of the factors you find willow in some commercial tea blends for menopause

Willow tea has been used to address joint pain and inflammation.

The bark from the willow contains salicin and is used to relieve headaches.

How to brew

Decoction: Add 1 heaped teaspoon of dried willow bark chips and 2 cup of cold water to a saucepan and bring to the boil and boil for 10 minutes. Remove from heat, cover and steep for 30 minutes. Consume.

This should leave you with one cup of willow tea.

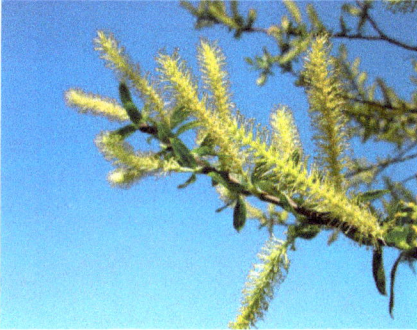

Do not use if pregnant or breastfeeding without the first consulting your health care professional. Willow bark may stop blood clotting do not use with blood thinning medication. Stop use 2 weeks before surgery.

Withania

Withania somnifera

Also known as Indian ginseng or Ashwagandha. Balance issues may be assisted using withania.

Withania leaf and root both are high in iron. Low iron is associated with feelings of fatigue, tiredness, anxious or depression. If this is you then withania may be worth including in your tea blend.

Studies have linked withania to lowering blood sugar and cortisol levels which may assist if you are feeling stressed. The root of the plant is believed to assist with memory.

Withania has the potential to increase libido for some women.

How to brew

Infusion: 1 teaspoon of dried leaf or 2-3 teaspoons of fresh leave per cup of boiling water. Steep 10 minutes.

Decoction: Add 2 teaspoons of dried root to 850 mls of cold water in a saucepan and boil for 15 minutes. Strain and consume.

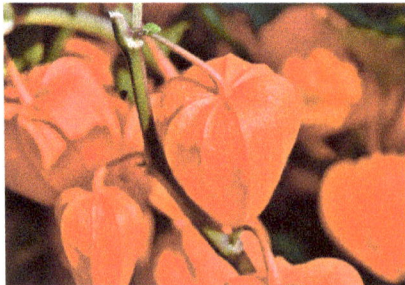

Do not use if pregnant or breastfeeding without the first consulting your health care professional. Do not use if you have an immune compromised condition or are on medication to suppress the immune system. Withania may lower blood pressure so check with your health care professional if you are on blood pressure medication or have a blood pressure issue. Do not use if you have a stomach ulcer.

Yarrow

Achillea millefolium

Here in Australia it is likely you have yarrow growing in your local park or perhaps even your yard. It is commonly found roadside or in unkempt fields. Of course, do ensure you have the correct plant when wild crafting.

For those women who seem to suffer from all the menopausal symptoms. Hot flushes, night sweats, digestive issues, vaginal irritation and discharge, sleep and anxiety issue. Yarrow is one of the herbs that may assist with the widest range of symptoms. While no herb is a 'cure all', Yarrow is a good choice to include in a general blend.

One to two cups a day is recommended.

How to brew

Infusion: 1 teaspoon of dried leaves or flowers or 1 tablespoon of fresh leaves and flowers per cup of boiling water. Steep for 10 minutes. Strain and consume. May be consumed cold.

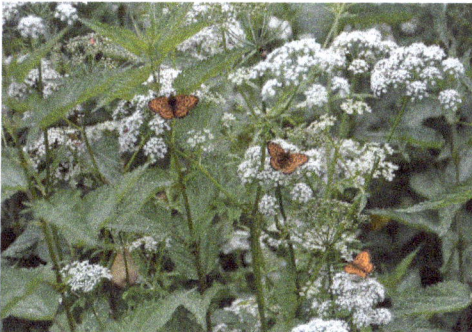

May slow blood clotting, if you have a blood disorder or are on medication for blood related issue please check with your health care provider before use. Stop using 2 weeks before surgery.

Yellow Dock

Rumex crispus

Yellow dock has laxative properties which are great if you are suffering from constipation.

Traditionally used to combat joint pain and **swelling associated with arthritis.**

Yellow dock contains iron, potassium, vitamin A and C which may be of assistance if your levels are low. Yellow dock is traditionally used for excessive menstrual bleeding.

How to brew

Infusion: 1 teaspoon of dried herb per cup of boiling water. Steep for 10 minutes.

Decoction: 1 tablespoon of fresh or dried root to 4 cups of cold water. Place in saucepan and bring to boil simmer for 15-20 minutes until you have 1 cup of liquid remaining. Decoction may be watered down and drunk throughout the day.

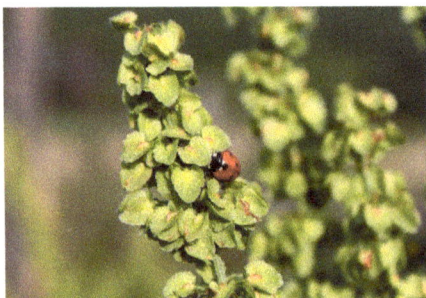

Do not eat yellow dock raw due to toxicity issues. Do not use if pregnant or breastfeeding. Do not use if you have blood disorders or are on blood thinning medication. Do not use if you have kidney or stomach issues or intestinal ulcers.

Zedoary

Curcuma zedoaria

Curcuma zerumbet

Sometimes referred to as white turmeric. Current thought is that zedoary helps with menstrual flow and thus, is not recommended for those women suffering from heavy menstrual bleeding.

Zedoary may assist with digestive issues. The consumption 30 minutes prior to meals is recommended.

It may possess aphrodisiac properties to assist both men and women. So if your sex drive is low this may be worth using.

How to brew

Infusion: 2 teaspoon of finely chopped root per cut of boiling water. Cover with a saucer or lid and Steep for 30 minutes. Strain and consume.

Decoction: Add 2 teaspoons of chopped root to your decoction blend.

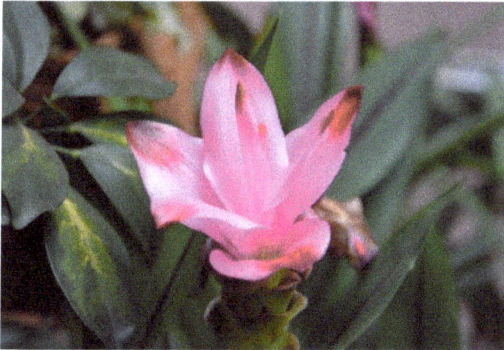

Do not use if pregnant. Seek advice from your health care professional before use in breast feeding. Zedoary is not well studied in humans, so information is limited.

Ziziphus

Ziziphus mauritiana

Also known as Jujube, ziziphus looks like a red date. If you are feeling moody, irritable, can't sleep or keep waking up then ziziphus may be great on its own or added to your blend.

May assist those women who are having digestive issues and constipation.

Ziziphus dates contain fibre, consumption may assist with constipation and weight loss. So, eat your ziziphus dates when you drink your tea ladies.

How to brew

Decoction: Use ¼ of a cup of dried fruit (dates) and two cups of cold water, place in a saucepan and bring to boil for 15 minutes. Strain and consume. Store remaining tea in the refrigerator and consume chilled or reheat if desired. Store for up to a week.

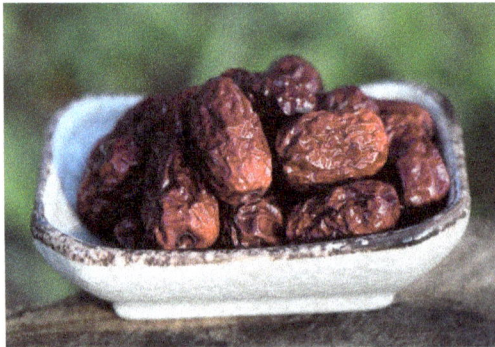

There is no information about safety of ziziphus for pregnancy or breast feeding, check with your health care professional before using. Diabetics' ziziphus may lower your blood sugar. Monitor and seek assistance if required. People who suffer from latex allergies are advised to avoid using ziziphus. Stop consumption two weeks before surgery.

Section 3

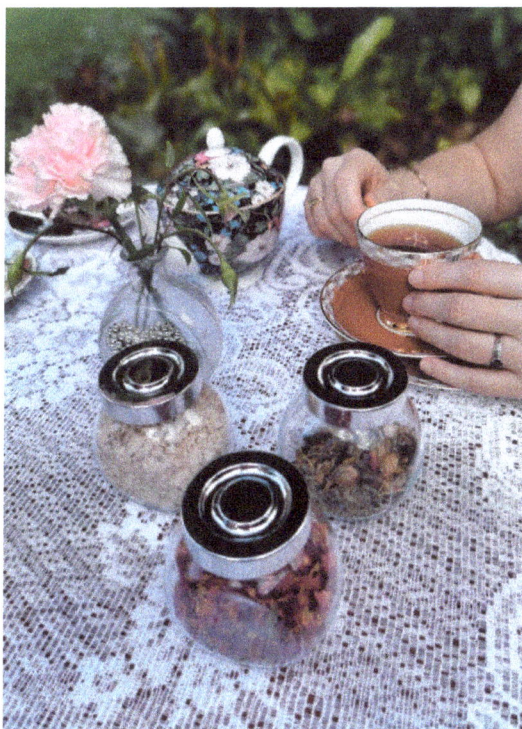

Tea Blends

Which tea should I Include in my blend?

Welcome to section three, by now you should understand how to make a cup of herbal tea both as an infusion and a decoction, the different in water temperature, kinds of teas and if you have read section two fully all the different teas that are available to assist the menopausal women.

Or maybe you have skimmed over section one and two and just want a quick answer to which teas may assist with yours or someone you know symptoms of menopause. Well you're in the right part of the book.

Once you have looked for the tea you think you will use it may be of benefit to go back and read each of the teas included in that blend so you have checked it is exactly what you want.

If you are buying a commercial tea blend you can use the second section to check if it has the herbs included to meet your requirements.

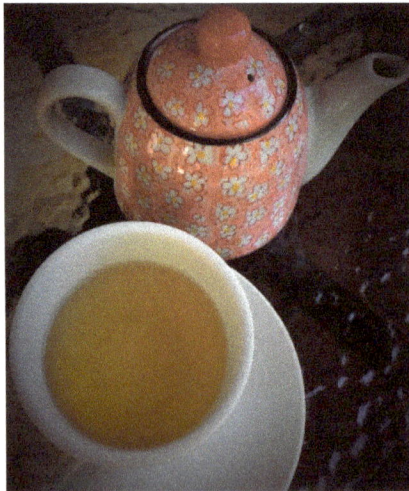

Tea for Menopause

Allergy tea blend may include:
Goldenrod, Hops, Kava, Lovage and Parsley.

Anxiety tea blend may include:
Valerian, Turmeric, Verbena, Wood betony, Yarrow, Ziziphus, Withania, Panax ginseng, Damiana, Echinacea, St Johns wort, Oat straw, Parsley, Passionflower, Rosemary, Saffron or Sage.

Bloating tea blend may include:
Thyme, Vitex, Nettle, Sarsaparilla, Sage, Kelp, Fennel, St John's Wort, Linden, Marjoram, Mistletoe, Hyssop, Lemon balm and Lemon verbena.

Body Odour tea blend may include:
Red clover, Sage, Rosemary and Oregano.

Breast Pain tea blend may include:
Red clover and Evening primrose.
Breast pain may be a symptom of a more serious condition please get it checked by a professional health care provider.

Brittle nail tea blend may include:
Raspberry leaf, Fennel seeds, Horsetail, Oat straw, Red clover, Alfalfa, Nettle, Dandelion. All have good levels of silica.

Dandelion, Rosehip and Chamomile, Mullein, Nettle and St Mary's thistle. All have zinc which is needed for nail and hair growth.

Burning tongue tea blend may include:
Chamomile
Avoid cinnamon and mint
Suggestion: may be beneficial to consume as iced tea.

Constipation tea blend may include:
Angelic, Fennel, Fenugreek, Flax, Hyssop, Kelp, Lemon verbena, Parsley, Rose, Moringa, Yellow dock, Senna and Ziziphus.

Depression tea blend may include:
Dill, Motherwort, Licorice, Kava, Rose, Roselle, Rosemary, Verbena, Panax ginseng, Red clover and Sage.

Difficulty concentrating tea blend may include:
Withania, Panax ginseng, Gotu Kola and St. Mary's thistle.

Digestive tea blend may include:
Catnip, Catuaba, Cinnamon, Chamomile, Ginger, Dill, Hawthorne, Holy basil, Hyssop, Lemon balm, Lemon verbena, Lemongrass, Licorice, Marigold/calendula, Marjoram, Meadowsweet, Oak Oregano, Roselle, Rosemary, Southernwood, Tarragon, Thyme, Wild yam, Yarrow and Zedoary.

Dizziness tea blend may include:
Withania, Peony, Betony and Cinnamon.

Fatigue tea blend may include:
Astragalus, Peony, Sarsaparilla, Tribulus, Ginseng, Rosehip, Gotu Kola, and Holy Basil.

Hair (thinning or loss) tea blend may include:
Nettle, Moringa, Saw Palmetto and Fennel.

Headache tea blend may include:
Betony, Lemon balm, Linden, Parsley, Peony, Moringa, Skullcap, Sarsaparilla, St John's Wort, Verbena, Willow, Yarrow.

Heavy bleeding tea blend may include:
Agrimony, Burnet, Plantain/Ribwort, Peony, Raspberry leaf, Rose, Angelica, Ginger, Cinnamon, Sage, Ladies Mantle and Vitex.

Tea for Menopause

Hot Flushes and Night Sweats tea blend may include:
Alfalfa, Angelica, Anise seed, Burnet, Caraway seed, Cinnamon, Damiana, Evening primrose, Fenugreek, Flaxseed, Ginger, Red clover, Sage, Hops, Licorice, Marigold/Calendula, Mint, Mistletoe, Mugwort, Passionflower, Roselle, Moringa, Solomons seal, St Mary's thistle, St John Wort, Tribulus, Turmeric, Valerian, Vitex, Wild yam, Yarrow and Ziziphus.

Hot Flushes and Night Sweats would be the most common symptom of menopause. There are more than twenty-five teas that may benefit those women experiencing these symptoms and if you consider the options to blend teas you have a huge selection to choose from. Sage in often used in a hot flush blend. As Sage is a bitter it may be good to combine it with other tea flavours you enjoy. Lavender, ginger, aniseed and licorice as well as mint are all able to impact the flavour.
If you have high blood pressure consider using passionflower, roselle, Solomons seal, turmeric and aniseed. If you have low blood pressure these may be best to avoid and licorice, ginger, parsley, vitex or ginseng may be a better choice for you. If your blood pressure is normal you can use whichever tea you chose.

Irritability tea blend may include:
Evening primrose, Lovage and Ziziphus.

Insomnia tea blend may include:
Catnip, Catuaba, Chamomile, Flaxseed, Heather, Hops, Lemon balm, Mistletoe, Motherwort, Nettle, Rosemary, Skullcap, Southernwood, St John's Wort, Thyme Valerian, Yarrow, and America ginseng.

Irregular heartbeat, palpitations tea blend may include:
Hawthorne, Licorice, Linden, Motherwort and Ziziphus.
If you are experiencing irregular heartbeat or palpitations please get it checked by your healthcare professional.

Irregular period's tea blend may include:
Angelica, Borage, Burnet, Mugwort and Peony.

Joint pains and aches tea blend may include:
Alfalfa, Fenugreek, Goldenrod, Holy Basil, Hydrangea, Kava, Kelp, Lemongrass, Marigold/Calendula, Meadowsweet, Mistletoe, Mullein, Nettle, Oat, Peony, Thyme, Turmeric, Vitex and Wild yam.

Tea for Menopause

Lack of Sleep tea blend may include:
Catnip, Fennel, Flaxseed, Kava, Lemon balm, Lovage, Nettle, Passionflower, Rosemary, Saffron, Tarragon, Thyme, Tribulus, Valerian, Vitex, Yarrow and Ziziphus.

Lack of Libido tea blend may include:
Betony, Catuaba, Damiana, Geranium, Hops, Moringa, Panax ginseng, Sarsaparilla, Summer savory, Turmeric, Withania and Zedoary.

Menstrual cramps tea blend may include:
Borage, Catnip, Cinnamon, Ginger, Dill, Horsetail, Hyssop, Lemon balm, Lemongrass, Licorice, Linden, Lovage, Motherwort, Mugwort, Nettle, Parsley, Passionflower, Peony, Red Clover, Raspberry leaf, Rose, Roselle, Saffron, Sage, Solomons seal, Southernwood, Verbena, Vitex, Willow and Yarrow.

Memory lapse tea blend may include:
Catuaba, Oat straw, Rosemary, Saffron, Sage, American ginseng.

Migraines tea blend may include:
Agrimony, Geranium, Lovage and Peony.

Mood swings tea blend may include:
Angelica, Catuaba, Cinnamon, Hops, Horse chestnut, Licorice, Lovage, Oat straw, Peony, Roselle, Skullcap, Solomons seal, and St John's Wort.

Muscle tension tea blend may include:
Anise seeds, Catnip, Hops, Kava, Motherwort, Mullein, Nettle, Parsley, Sarsaparilla and Yarrow.

Nausea tea blend may include:
Ginger, Lemon balm, Lemongrass, Nettle and Summer savory.

Stress tea blend may include:
Borage, Catnip, Catuaba, Geranium, Holy basil, Hops, Lemon balm, Licorice, Linden, Mugwort, Oat straw, Tarragon, Valerian, Panax ginseng, and Ziziphus.

Sugar craving tea blend may include:
Cinnamon, Ginger, Jasmine and Withania.

Urinary tract infection tea blend may include:
Betony, Chamomile, Echinacea, Damiana, Goldenrod, Heather, Horsetail, Hydrangea, Hyssop, Lovage, Meadowsweet, Nettle, Oregano, Parsley, Rose, Southernwood, Turmeric, Bearberry and Yarrow.

Vaginal dryness tea blend may include:
Damiana, Dill, Hops, Nettle, Saw Palmetto and Solomons seal.

Vaginal discharge tea blend may include:
Agrimony, Nettle, Oregano, Peony, Turmeric and Yarrow.

Vaginal Irritation tea blend may include:
Bearberry, Dill, Hops, Nettle, Peony, Saw Palmetto, Solomons seal, and Turmeric.

Weight loss for menopausal women tea blend may include:
Damian, Devils claw, Jasmine, Kelp, Lemongrass, Sage, Turmeric and Ziziphus.

The maths of tea options.

Excluding lemon, lime and orange which we will consider an additive, this book contains the details of 102 herbal teas which gives you the following possibilities:

1 tea used to make a cup of tea is 102 different varieties.
2 tea blends is 5,151.
3 tea blends is 171,700.
4 tea blends is 4,249,575.
5 tea blends is 83,291,670.

Which gives you the choice of 87,718,198 different tea combination to assist you as you transition through your menopausal journey. What a wonderful variety is there for our choosing.

Ladies it's time for tea!

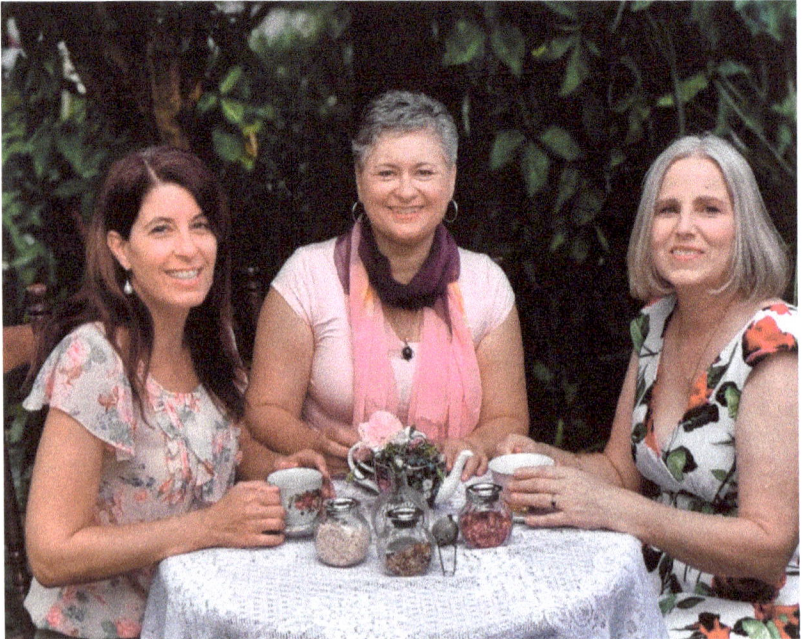

My favourite tea blends

My menopausal story

Tea for Menopause

My menopausal story.

Tea for Menopause

My favourite tea blends.

Tea for Menopause

Acknowledgement of photos

Front cover: Mary-Leigh Scheerhoorn

Page 3 Lady on swing: JL G from Pixabay.

Page 6 Tea Party: Mary-Leigh Scheerhoorn.

Page 9 Tea Party: Mary-Leigh Scheerhoorn.

Page 11 tea with iPad: rawpixel from Pixabay.

Page 15 teas: gate74 from Pixabay.

Page 17 Storage: Mathias Megerle from Pixabay.

Page 19. Beverage: Clker-Free-Vector_Images from Pixabay.

Page 20 tea ball: Bruno Glatsch from Pixabay.

Page 21 decoction: vivi14216 from Pixabay.

Page 22 Additives: Myshun from Pixabay.

Page 23 ice flowers: rawpixel from Pixabay.

Page 24 Teas: Mary-Leigh Scheerhoorn.

Page 25 Tea party: Mary Leigh Scheerhoorn.

Herb photos

Agrimony: Richard Revel from Pixabay.

Alfalfa: James C from Pixabay

Angelica: anandasandra from Pixabay.

Anise seeds: Wolfgang Eckert from Pixabay.

Astragalus: Marc Miraille from Pixabay

Bearberry: rmadison from Pixabay.

Betony: Rhiannon from Pixabay.

Borage: Araneel from Pixabay.

Burnet: Stan1952 from Pixabay.

Calendula: Marina Pershina from Pixabay.

Caraway seed: David Mark from Pixabay.

Catnip: rebeck96 from Pixabay.

Catuaba Bark: Klimkin from Pixabay.

Chamomile: cocoparisienne from Pixabay.

Cinnamon: Leone from Pixabay.

Damiana: Albert Dezetter from Pixabay.

Devil's claw: Kyra Howearth.

Dill: pgbkr from Pixabay.

Echinacea: Sonja Kalee from Pixabay.

Evening Primrose: Hans Benn from Pixabay.

Fennel: Beverly Barkley from Pixabay.

Fenugreek: Sandeep Handa from Pixabay.

Flaxseed: alexdante from Pixabay.

Geranium: WikimediaImages from Pixabay.

Ginger: Mary-Leigh Scheerhoorn.

Ginseng: whaltns17 from Pixabay and Bosmin Kang from Pixabay.

Goldenrod: Hans Benn from Pixabay.

Gotu kola: Beverly Buckley from Pixabay.

Hawthorne: Hans Braxmeir from Pixabay.

Heather: Filip Kruchlik from Pixabay.

Hollyhock: Ben Lesure from Pixabay.

Holly Basil: Anita Williams.

Hops: moritz320 from Pixabay.

Horsetail: Susanne Jutzeler, suju-foto from Pixabay.

Hydrangea: Pexels from Pixabay.

Hyssop: Sonja Rieck from Pixabay.

Jasmine: Laana13 from Pixabay.

Kava: Radek Spata from Pixabay.

Kelp: bluebudgie from Pixabay.

Lavender: Braxmeier from Pixabay.

Lemon and Lime: Mary-Leigh Scheerhoorn.

Lemon balm: Congerdesign from Pixabay.

Lemon grass: Bishnu Sarangi from Pixabay.

Lemon verbane: Lebensmittelfotos from Pixabay.

Licorice: Mary-Leigh Scheerhoorn

Tea for Menopause

Linden: Inga Zvaigzne from Pixabay.

Lovage: Marketa Machova from Pixabay.

Marjoram: Marketa Machova from Pixabay.

Marshmallow: Couleur from Pixabay.

Meadowsweet: Jeon Sang-O from Pixabay.

Mint: Congerdesign from Pixabay.

Mistletoe: Simy27 from Pixabay.

Moringa: Iskandar. Ab. Rashid from Pixabay.

Motherwort: Norma Jones from Pixabay.

Mugwort: Merja Partanen from Pixabay.

Mullein: Marketa Machova from Pixabay

Nettle: AllNikArt from Pixabay.

Oak: Manfred Antranias Zimmer from Pixabay

Oats: Jan Nijman from Pixabay.

Orange peel: GimpWorkshop from Pixabay.

Oregano: ariesa66 from Pixabay.

Parsley: AllNikArt from Pixabay.

Passionflower: Richard Revel from Pixabay.

Pau D'arco: Anita Williams

Peony: Lee seonghak from Pixabay/

Plantain: WikimediaImages from Pixabay.

Raspberry leaf: Miklos Kocsis from Pixabay.

Red Clover: Couleur from Pixabay.

Rose: Mary-Leigh Scheerhoorn and Anita Williams.

Roselle: JoaKwan from Pixabay.

Rosemary: andreas N from Pixabay.

Saffron: Marc Pascual from Pixabay.

Sage: Marc Pascual from Pixabay.

Sarsaparilla: Marc Pascual from Pixabay.

Saw palmetto: JoaoBOliver from Pixabay.

Sea buckthorn: Leo Ainsalo from Pixabay.

Senna: HOervin56 from Pixabay.

Sheep's Sorrel: Constanze Riechert-Kurtze from Pixabay.

Shepherd's purse: Alesancra Bolovenco from Pixabay.

Skullcap: ustalij_pony. from Pixabay.

Solomons seal: Jurgen Koditz from Pixabay.

Southernwood: Kyra Howearth.

St John's Wort: Vasil Stefanov from Pixabay.

St Mary's thistle. Celia Lepelletier from Pixabay.

Summer Savory: Hans Braxmeier from Pixabay

Tarragon: Nathan Elliot from Pixabay/

Thyme: Th G from Pixabay.

Tribulus: Anita Williams

Turmeric: Steve Buissinne from Pixabay.

Valerian: LoggaWiggler from Pixabay.

Verbena: Kerstin Riemer from Pixabay.

Vitex: daynaw3390 from Pixabay.

Wild Yam: Jan Haerer from Pixabay.

Willow: WikimediaImages from Pixabay.

Withania: Capri23auto from Pixabay.

Yarrow: PublicDomainPictures from Pixabay.

Yellow dock: Emilian Robert Vicol from Pixabay.

Zedoary: JacLou DL from Pixabay.

Ziziphus: SW Yang from Pixabay.

Section 3: Mary-Leigh Scheerhoorn

Tea: Anita Williams

Tea party: Meg Cartwright.